RACING WEIGHT

QUICK START GUIDE

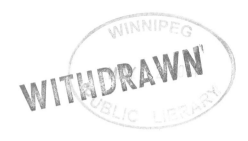

RACING WEIGHT

QUICK START GUIDE

A 4-Week Weight-Loss Plan for Endurance Athletes

Matt Fitzgerald

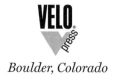

VELO press

Boulder, Colorado

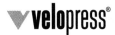

3002 Sterling Circle, Suite 100
Boulder, Colorado 80301-2338 USA
(303) 440-0601 · Fax (303) 444-6788 · E-mail velopress@competitorgroup.com

Distributed in the United States and Canada by Ingram Publisher Services

Library of Congress Cataloging-in-Publication Data
Fitzgerald, Matt.
Racing weight quick start guide: a 4-week weight-loss plan for endurance athletes / Matt Fitzgerald.
  p. cm.
Includes bibliographical references and index.
ISBN 978-1-934030-72-1 (pbk.: alk. paper)
1. Endurance sports—Training. 2. Endurance sports—Physiological aspects. 3. Athletes—Nutrition. 4. Body weight—Regulation. I. Title.
GV749.5.F59 2010
613.2'024796—dc22

                                                    2010043661

For information on purchasing VeloPress books, please call (800) 811-4210, ext. 2138, or visit www.velopress.com.

Editorial production by *Marrathon* Production Services. www.marrathon.net
Cover design by *the*BookDesigners
Cover photo by Brad Kaminski
Interior design by Katie Jennings
Illustrations by Kagan McLeod
Composition by Lisa Liddy, The Printed Page

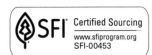

15   14   13   /   4   5   6   7   8   9   10

CONTENTS

ACKNOWLEDGMENTS

I wish to express my heartfelt gratitude to the following people, without whose help and support this book would not be what it is: John Berardi, Ted Costantino, Fred Duffner, Nataki Fitzgerald, Sean Fitzgerald, Megan Forbes, Jade Hays, Renee Jardine, Asker Jeukendrup, Lina Konner, William Lunn, Christine Marra, Robert Portman, and Dave Trendler.

INTRODUCTION

The relationship between power output and body weight is every-thing in the sport of cycling. This relationship, known as the power-to-weight ratio, is the single best predictor of a cyclist's race performance capacity. Power produced by the cyclist's body moves the bike forward. The weight of the cyclist's body resists for-ward movement. So the more a cyclist can increase his power output at any given weight and the more he can reduce his body weight with-out sacrificing power output, the better he can perform on the bike.

The same principle applies in running and other endurance sports. While it is not possible to accurately measure power output in these other sports, different measurements tell the same story. For example, VO_2 max, or the maximum rate of oxygen consumption, can be used as a rough proxy for power-to-weight ratio in runners. Just as bigger cyclists can generate more power than smaller ones, bigger runners can consume more oxygen (which drives muscle contractions and forward movement) than smaller ones. But VO_2max as we know it is adjusted for body weight. So, while a 200-lb. jogger might have more absolute aerobic power than a 120-lb. elite marathoner, the latter is able to consume much more oxygen per kilogram of body mass. The elite marathoner's VO_2max will be significantly higher, and that is the stat that matters for performance. VO_2max predicts running performance (and rowing performance, cross-country skiing performance, etc.) as well as power-to-weight ratio predicts cycling performance. There are two ways you can increase your VO_2max:

- Increase your aerobic capacity with training
- Lose weight without losing aerobic capacity

In 2009, researchers at Southern Connecticut State University conducted an interesting study in which they compared the effects of sprint interval training (a good way to increase power capacity), weight loss, and a combination of sprint interval training and weight loss on the power-to-weight ratio of experienced cyclists.[1] Thirty-four cyclists, separated into four groups, participated in the study. For 10 weeks, one group added twice-weekly sprint interval sessions to their training while maintaining their current body weight; a second group continued with their normal training while actively pursuing weight loss through dieting; a third group added sprint intervals and pursued weight loss; and a fourth "control" group continued with their normal training and maintained their current body weight.

The results were telling. Members of the sprint interval–training group improved their power-to-weight ratio by 10 percent, on average. They achieved this gain entirely through an increase in their power output, as their weight did not change. Members of the weight-loss group increased their power-to-weight ratio almost as much—by an average 9.3 percent. This gain was achieved entirely through weight loss (they lost 11 lbs. on average), as their power output did not change. As you might expect, members of the control group experienced no

1 W. R. Lunn, J. A. Finn, and R. S. Axtell, "Effects of Sprint Interval Training and Body-Weight Reduction on Power to Weight Ratio in Experienced Cyclists," *Journal of Strength and Conditioning Research* 23, no. 4 (July 2009): 1217–24.

gain in power, no weight loss, and thus no change in power-to-weight ratio. But what might surprise you is that members of the combined sprint interval–training and weight-loss group also did not improve their power-to-weight ratio over the 10-week study period. The problem for this group was that, while they did lose a significant amount of weight through dietary restriction, this very restriction seemed to prevent them from gaining any power through sprint interval training. More specifically, suggested the authors of the study, inadequate protein intake kept their muscles from adapting to the stress imposed by the sprints.

The general conclusion the authors drew from the results of their investigation was that cyclists seeking to enhance their power-to-weight ratio should *either* add sprint intervals to their training *or* lose weight, but should not do both simultaneously. This conclusion is consistent with the observation of many other exercise scientists, coaches, and athletes that the aggressive pursuit of weight loss through dietary restriction is not compatible with aggressive training for maximum performance. Maximum weight loss and maximum performance cannot be equal priorities for an endurance athlete at any given time.

The truth of this point becomes even clearer when you consider the fastest possible way to safely lose weight: the very-low-calorie diet (VLCD). Medical professionals sometimes place severely obese patients on a diet of just 800 calories per day when the health effects of their body weight are considered to constitute an emergency requiring immediate and drastic correction. A modest 800 calories per day is about the minimum amount of food energy a severely obese person requires to keep all of his or her vital organs functioning properly. On a VLCD a patient can expect to lose three to five pounds per week. It is the fastest possible way to safely lose weight.

Very-low-calorie diets are sometimes combined with light exercise to promote additional weight loss. Long or intense workouts are not possible on such a diet, however. Muscle energy supplies plummet if you are eating only 800 calories a day, leaving your muscles incapable of vigorous or sustained work. Imagine trying to perform your normal endurance training on a VLCD. Forget about it! Your workouts would be complete disasters and you would lose fitness as quickly as you lost fat.

Because body weight has a major effect on endurance sports performance, competitive endurance athletes should do all they can to shed any excess fat they might carry on their bodies. But since the goal is performance, endurance athletes cannot pursue weight loss through high levels of caloric restriction that leave their muscles improperly fueled for training—at least not when they are actively seeking to maximize their fitness for racing.

I made this point previously in my book *Racing Weight: How to Get Lean for Peak Performance*. The primary objective of that book was to show endurance athletes how to shed excess body fat in a way that complemented rather than compromised their efforts to train for peak fitness. For this reason, none of the five steps in my Racing Weight plan entailed drastically cutting calories from the athlete's diet. It is possible and appropriate to pursue weight loss more aggressively when maximizing race fitness is not an immediate goal, and *Racing Weight* offered general guidelines for faster weight loss. Many of the book's readers requested more detailed guidelines for faster weight loss. I told them I left those guidelines out of the first book in order to leave room for a sequel.

But, honestly, the real reason is this: I deemed it important to steer endurance athletes out of that mindset. I saw too many endurance athletes trying to lose weight on the same crash diets couch potatoes use, thereby sabotaging their own training and racing. I felt that the resource endurance athletes most needed was one that would help them lose weight gradually and steadily while building competitive fitness.

While there is a time and a place for endurance athletes to seek faster weight loss, the most popular weight-loss diets are no more appropriate for endurance athletes in that circumstance than in any other. An endurance athlete who chooses to pursue fast weight loss outside of a race-focused training cycle must do so with his or her race objectives in mind. Even as the athlete reduces calories to promote fat loss, he or she must perform the necessary training to prepare for the race-focused buildup to come and therefore must fuel himself or herself in a way that supports that training. The athlete needs an integrated nutrition and training plan that balances quick weight loss with appropriate "off-season" or "pre-base" fitness development. Following the Atkins Diet or going on a juice fast and putting training on the back burner won't cut it.

The main purpose of the *Racing Weight Quick Start Guide* is to fill the gap left by its predecessor. The heart of this book is a set of integrated nutrition and training plans specifically designed to help endurance athletes lose fat quickly before they embark on race-focused training.

Whether you're a cyclist, a runner, or a triathlete, whether you have a lot of weight to lose or just a little, whether you're a recreational athlete or a hardcore competitor, there's a plan here for you.

Here's what to expect. In Chapter 1, I will present a step-by-step explanation of how to estimate your racing weight. This method might not yield a 100 percent accurate prediction of your ideal racing weight, but it will give you a sensible goal to pursue and provide information to help you choose the right quick start plan for your needs. Chapter 2 reviews the five steps of the Racing Weight system— improving your diet quality, balancing your energy sources, nutrient timing, managing your appetite, and training for racing weight. Chapter 3 provides an overview of the quick start plans. It explains how each of the five components of the Racing Weight system is practiced somewhat differently during a four- to eight-week quick start plan than it is within a race-focused training cycle. The remaining chapters provide the meal plans and training plans you will need to execute your quick start.

The plans in this book are like no weight-loss programs you have encountered before. Your quick start plan combines the objectives

▶ ATHLETES NEED AN INTEGRATED NUTRITION AND TRAINING PLAN THAT BALANCES QUICK WEIGHT LOSS WITH APPROPRIATE "OFF-SEASON" OR "PRE-BASE" FITNESS DEVELOPMENT.

of rapid short-term weight loss and foundational fitness development for endurance racing. This is exactly the right combination for an endurance athlete who is just returning to training after an off-season break or just starting out. As in the Racing Weight plan itself, there is no shtick or novelty element involved. Both the dietary and training prescriptions are based on sound science—like the study of athletes described earlier—and the proven practices of the world's best coaches and athletes. I am confident that whichever plan you choose to follow will move you a big step closer to your optimal racing weight and toward achieving your goals and dreams as an athlete.

TARGETING YOUR RACING WEIGHT

What is racing weight? I define it simply as the combined body weight and body composition (or body-fat percentage) associated with an endurance athlete's peak performance level. The most important thing to understand about racing weight is that it is defined functionally, not theoretically. When you are in the best racing shape you can possibly attain, you are at your ideal racing weight. It doesn't matter if that weight (and body-fat percentage) is higher or lower than you might expect or some formula might predict. Performance decides your true racing weight.

The second most important thing to understand about racing weight is that it is not all about body weight. In fact, the body-weight component is secondary to the body-composition component. This is true because any given athlete often can attain a desired weight, but at a variety of different body-fat percentages. Only when that weight is attained in conjunction with a minimal body-fat percentage will the athlete be capable of peak racing performance.

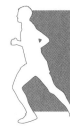

> ► ANY CHANGE IN YOUR WEIGHT OR BODY-FAT PERCENTAGE THAT NEGATIVELY AFFECTS YOUR PERFORMANCE IS A BAD THING.

Racing weight is different from healthy weight. Each person has a fairly broad "healthy weight range" and can have more or less optimal health anywhere within that range. With the exception of some swimmers and heavyweight rowers, most endurance athletes achieve their best race performances when their weight is near the bottom of their personal healthy weight range, provided this weight is achieved through proper training and diet. This is true primarily because extra body weight increases the energy cost of movement. Body fat is the primary source of excess weight in most endurance athletes. Research has consistently shown that the best endurance athletes have the leanest body compositions. Not every athlete can get as lean as the world's best, but every endurance athlete is at his best when he's close to his personal leanest. The most significant change most endurance athletes experience in moving closer to their racing weight is a loss of body fat.

There is such a thing as being too light or too lean for maximum race performance. It's a state that some endurance athletes end up in when they lose sight of the fact that performance defines ideal weight and not the other way around. The surest way to avoid becoming too light or lean is to eat and train expressly for performance rather than weight loss, trusting that appropriate fat loss will occur as your performance improves. Consistently monitoring your performance in training acts as a check against going off track. Any change in your weight or body-fat percentage that negatively affects your performance is a bad thing.

It is acceptable to make short-term exceptions to the principle of prioritizing performance over weight loss. That's what a quick start period is for. But even during a quick start, when fat loss becomes the highest priority, performance remains the ultimate end. The training and nutrition practices that constitute a quick start are designed not only to yield rapid fat loss but also to create a solid foundation for future performance.

When I speak about weight management for endurance athletes, I often ask those in the audience who know their ideal racing weight to raise their hands. There are always a few. When I select an athlete to tell me how he or she knows his or her racing weight, the answer is always the same: through experience. There can be no other answer because there is no other way to definitively determine one's racing weight. A typical case is that of my colleague Mario Fraioli, a runner with a 5,000 meter personal best of 14:30. He knows his racing weight is 136 lbs. because he has raced at that weight, at lower weights, and at higher weights, and he consistently performs best at or very near 136.

In the total population of endurance athletes, for every Mario Fraioli there are several athletes who do not know their racing weight because they have good reason to believe they have never reached it. How do you know if you have never reached your racing weight? You can make this judgment on the basis of some commonsense indicators:

- You weigh significantly more now than you did in your younger days.
- You have a lot of visible excess body fat.
- You are new enough to your sport to know you haven't yet come close to having your best race.

Very few of us need anyone's help in figuring out we could stand to lose some weight, even if it's mainly for the purpose of racing faster.

A more rigorous way to determine if you are above your ideal racing weight is to have your body-fat percentage measured and compare it against the ideal racing weight body-fat percentage range for your age and gender. If you're above that range, you're above your racing weight.

If you have not yet reached your racing weight and therefore don't know it, you could benefit from a reliable method of estimating your racing weight. If nothing else, such an estimate would provide a goal for you. Again, there is no such thing as a scientifically accurate racing-weight calculator, but there is a method you can use to create an estimated racing weight that can serve as an initial goal.

This method relies heavily on body-fat measurements because it's really your optimal body-fat percentage that determines your ideal racing weight. While age, gender, genes, and other factors limit how much you can reduce your body-fat percentage, proper training and nutrition will help you get it down to a level far below the average for the general population. Researchers have gathered solid evidence of the body-fat percentages generally attainable for different age and gender groups, and scientists have identified certain factors that make these optimal body-fat percentages more or less attainable. On the basis of this knowledge, it is possible to make a realistic prediction as to how much any given athlete can lower his or her body-fat percentage. This prediction in turn can be used to generate an estimated racing weight for the individual.

Estimating your individual racing weight begins with a realistic prediction of how much you can lower your body-fat percentage.

BEFORE YOU STEP ON A BODY-FAT SCALE

HERE ARE SOME USAGE GUIDELINES THAT APPLY TO MOST BODY-FAT SCALES:

- Always measure your body fat at the same time of day, preferably at least two hours after eating.

- Make sure you are well hydrated.

- Use the bathroom before stepping on the scale.

- Moisten a towel and step on it with bare feet before stepping on the scale (to enhance conductivity).

- Make sure the scale is on a flat, hard surface (such as bathroom tiles).

- If you have a good reason to believe that your body-fat percentage is already low (e.g., you have visible abdominal musculature), purchase a scale with an "athletic" mode. Scales without this feature are less accurate for lean individuals.

CONDUCT A BODY-FAT TEST

To generate an estimate of your optimal performance weight you will need to start by getting an initial body-fat measurement. The easiest and most affordable way to measure your body-fat percentage (but not the most accurate) is to step on a body-fat scale. But there are other methods. The most accurate is DEXA scanning, which you may be familiar with as the method physicians use to measure bone density. The disadvantage of this method is that the testing is expensive and not widely available, so it's not a method that most athletes can use to regularly track changes in their body composition. Hydrostatic weighing, or dunking, once known as the gold-standard method of body-fat measurement, suffers from the same disadvantages and is not as accurate as DEXA scanning. The most popular do-it-yourself method of body-fat testing before the advent of the body-fat scale was the skinfold caliper method, but this requires training and practice to do correctly and is no more accurate even when done correctly.

Table 1.1 presents body-fat percentage ranges associated with ideal racing weights in men and women of different ages. In other words, it shows the body-fat ranges of men and women of different ages who have attained peak fitness through optimal training and diet. For example, women between the ages of 30 and 39 who train and eat right long enough to attain a lifetime peak race-fitness level typically have body-fat percentages between 11 and 17 percent. But there are individual variations within this range. Those with genes favoring lean body composition, who have never put on substantial excess body fat, and who train maximally for their sport will have body-fat levels closer to 11 percent. Those without genes favoring lean body composition, who have put on excess body fat in the past, and who do not train maximally for their sport will have body-fat levels closer to 17 percent. But that's still pretty low.

TABLE 1.1 IDEAL RACING WEIGHT BODY-FAT RANGES

MEN				WOMEN			
20–29	30–39	40–49	50+	20–29	30–39	40–49	50+
3–10%	5–12%	6–15%	8–17%	10–16%	11–17%	13–20%	14–22%

DEFINE YOUR GOAL BODY-FAT PERCENTAGE

Use your initial body-fat measurement and Table 1.1 to make a realistic prediction of the body-fat percentage you are likely to have in a state of lifetime peak fitness. If your current body-fat percentage is substantially outside the range for your gender and age group, then your initial goal should be to get your body-fat percentage down to the upper limit of your range. For example, if you are a 49-year-old man and your current body-fat percentage is 25, your initial goal should be to get it down to 15 percent, which represents the upper limit of the 6 to 15 percent ideal racing weight body-fat percentage range of men between the ages of 40 and 49 years. You may eventually be able to get it lower, but you might not. It's especially difficult for those who are substantially overweight to know how lean they can ultimately get because in some members of this population a certain amount of excess fat accumulation is irreversible and in others it's not. So if you are substantially overweight, it's best to set a safe target in the beginning. That said, 15 percent body fat is a very lean body composition for a 49-year-old man and represents a more aggressive target than most physicians would give an overweight patient of that age.

If your current body-fat level is close to the upper limit of the range for your gender and age or already within that range, then your target body-fat percentage should be based on how much room for improvement there is in your current diet and fitness level. The more drastically you plan to improve your diet and increase your training load, starting today, in the pursuit of peak fitness, the more you can expect to reduce your body-fat percentage. The better your current diet is and the closer you are to peak fitness already, the less change you can expect in your body-fat percentage.

For example, suppose you are a 24-year-old woman with a body-fat percentage of 23 who lives on fast food and is returning to cycling after a long layoff. You plan to clean up your diet and gradually build your training load to the level it was at when you competed in the past. Therefore, you can expect to reduce your body-fat percentage quite a bit, perhaps down to the middle of your ideal range of 10 to 16 percent. Now let's assume you are a 33-year-old man with a current body-fat percentage of 14; you consider your diet already very healthy and you are returning to triathlon training after a short break that followed a personal best Ironman 70.3 race. In this case you can expect to reduce your body-fat percentage only a little in tidying up your diet that last little bit and returning to peak fitness. Perhaps you can get it down to 10.5 percent.

If your current body-fat percentage is outside your ideal range by 10 percent or more, it's best to set an intermediate or stepping-stone goal instead of aiming directly for the upper limit of your ideal range. In this circumstance, getting all the way from your current body-fat percentage to your ultimate goal will take long enough that you'll need the motivation provided by an intermediate target. I recommend that you begin with closing the gap between your current body-fat percentage and the upper limit of your ideal body-fat percentage range by splitting the difference. For example, suppose you are a 35-year-old male whose current body fat percentage is 26. That's 14 percent above the upper limit of 12 percent for your age group's ideal range. Half the difference between 26 percent and 12 percent is 7 percent. Thus, your intermediate goal should be to reduce your body fat to 19 percent (half the difference plus the upper limit, or 12+7). Getting

▶ OLDER ATHLETES SHOULD FIND IT NO MORE CHALLENGING TO REACH THEIR IDEAL RANGE THROUGH THE QUICK START AND RACING WEIGHT METHODS THAN YOUNGER ATHLETES.

all the way down to 12 percent is probably an attainable long-term goal, but aiming for it directly might lead to frustration, as it will take many months to get there.

Many people find it more difficult to lose weight as they get older. This may have less to do with age itself than with the effects of body fat accumulation over time, muscle loss, and declining activity levels on metabolism. Research has generally shown that older persons experience the same improvements in body composition as younger persons in response to exercise and calorie restriction. Older persons cannot get quite as lean as younger persons due to the irreversible accumulation of fat around the internal organs, a reality that is accounted for in the ideal body fat percentage ranges presented in Table 1.1 (see page 12). But if you are an older athlete you should find it no more challenging to reach your ideal range through the quick start and Racing Weight methods than a younger athlete will find reaching his or her lower ideal range.

Does this approach to setting body composition goals sound a bit like guesswork? It is to some degree. But it's the best we can do. And they are not wild guesses. If you follow the structure I've provided and use your God-given reasoning faculties, you can come up with a personal target that is very appropriate.

One other guideline I can give you that will help you make good guesses is this: Don't aim for the very bottom end of your gender and age-group range unless you are naturally lean (that is, if you naturally put on fat slowly and lose it easily) and plan to train maximally for your sport.

Maximal training means doing the maximum amount of training beneficial to the athlete without consideration of schedule constraints or personal preferences. Few endurance athletes are willing and able to train maximally for their sport. And the difference between maximal training and the amount of training the average endurance athlete is willing and able to do is enough to make a significant difference in terms of what body-fat percentage is realistic. For example, a triathlete for whom 25 hours of training per week would be maximal but who actually trains 15 hours per week cannot expect to get his body-fat percentage down quite as low as if he did train maximally.

Keep this in mind when predicting your racing-weight body-fat percentage. If you are unwilling or unable to train maximally for your sport, don't aim for the lower limit of the racing-weight body-fat percentage range that applies to your age group.

CALCULATING YOUR WEIGHT LOSS

The final step in determining your racing weight is to calculate how much weight—more specifically *fat*—you will have to lose to get down to your goal body-fat percentage. Let's look at how to do this with an example.

Let's say you are a 38-year-old female who weighs 140 lbs. and has 22 percent body fat. Your diet is already very clean, but you have always had great difficulty shedding excess body fat. Therefore you decide to make a conservative racing weight estimate, at least to start with. Your initial goal is to get down to 17 percent body fat (the upper limit of your ideal range) through improved training and diet. Here's how to calculate how much you will weigh when you get your body-fat percentage down to that level.

STEP 1: CALCULATE YOUR BODY-FAT MASS

To do this, you multiply your current weight by your body-fat percentage.

In this example, 140 lbs. x 0.22 = 30.8 lbs.

Body fat mass = current weight x current body-fat percentage

STEP 2: CALCULATE YOUR LEAN BODY MASS

To find this number, subtract your fat mass from your current weight. In this example, 140 lbs. – 30.8 lbs. = 109.2 lbs.

Lean body mass = current weight – fat mass

STEP 3: CALCULATE YOUR GOAL WEIGHT

First find your goal lean-body-mass percentage by subtracting your goal body-fat percentage from 100. Now express this number as a percentage, or in decimal form. In this example, 100 − 17 = 83 leaves our athlete with an 83 percent goal lean body mass.

Now to find your goal weight, divide your current lean body mass (found in step 2) by your goal lean body mass percentage (as you just calculated). In this example, 109.2 ÷ 0.83 = 131.6.

Goal weight = current lean body mass ÷ goal-lean-body-mass percentage

There you have it: an imperfect but reliable method to estimate your racing weight (and body-fat percentage). It is not a 100 percent accurate prediction in most cases, but it is accurate enough to serve its purpose of giving you a solid goal to aim for in your quick start and beyond as you follow the Racing Weight system to train and fuel your way toward peak fitness.

THE RACING
WEIGHT SYSTEM

The two simplest ways to lose weight are to eat less and exercise more. But the simplest ways to lose weight are not always the best and most effective ways. Substantially reducing food intake typically causes persistent hunger, which most people cannot put up with for very long. And for endurance athletes, cutting way back on calories is likely to sabotage performance by causing muscle wasting and muscle fuel depletion. Exercising more is always a good idea for the sedentary person seeking to lose weight, but it is not always smart for the competitive endurance athlete. Your training volume should be determined strictly by your performance objectives. It is unwise to increase your training beyond the level judged appropriate to maximize your performance for the sake of losing more weight because your performance would inevitably suffer.

So how should you pursue weight loss as an endurance athlete? The Racing Weight system consists of five specific measures you can take as an athlete to attain your optimal body weight and body composition for performance:

1. Improve your diet quality.

2. Balance your energy sources.

3. Time nutrients.

4. Manage your appetite.

5. Train for racing weight.

The Racing Weight approach doesn't require a conscious reduction in food intake or an unnecessary increase in training load, so you can consistently practice all these measures whenever you are actively training for races.

When you are not actively training for races, you can, and in some instances should, pursue weight loss somewhat differently. A quick start is a short period preceding a cycle of race-focused training in which fast weight loss becomes your primary immediate goal. The five fundamentals of the Racing Weight system still apply, but how they play out in meals and training is a little different. If you've already read *Racing Weight*, you can skip ahead to Chapter 3 to see how each principle works within the quick start plan.

IMPROVING YOUR DIET QUALITY

It doesn't take a PhD in nutrition to improve your diet quality. Most of us have a basic understanding of which foods are high quality and which are low quality. American elite cyclist Chris Horner knew that the fast food meals, candy bars, and soft drinks in his diet were low quality and the fruits and vegetables he was not eating were high quality. So when he set about improving his diet for the 2009 season, he reduced his consumption of the former and increased his consumption of the latter. Nothing to it.

Improving diet quality in this informal way can be tricky, though, because research has shown that most of us think we eat better than we really do. That's why I created the Diet Quality Score (DQS), a simple tool that allows athletes to quantify the quality of their diet. The DQS makes the process of improving diet quality easier and more reliable because with it you can determine exactly how close to perfect your diet has to be for you to attain your racing weight. Just calculate the DQS of your current diet, then continue to calculate it day by day as you make changes to it. When you attain your racing weight, take note of your DQS and try to maintain it at that level.

In the DQS system, foods are classified in 11 categories. There are six categories of high-quality foods that add points to your daily score: fruit, vegetables, whole grains, lean proteins, low-fat dairy, and essential fatty acids. On the other hand, five categories of low-quality foods that subtract points from your daily score: refined grains, sweets, fried foods, whole-milk dairy, and fatty proteins. Table 2.1 presents these categories in more detail.

Calculating your DQS is similar to counting calories, but far more easy. Just note how many portions of each type of food listed in Table 2.2 you eat during a given day. Assign the appropriate number of points based on how many servings of each type of food you eat. You'll notice that some foods lose value the more often you eat them in a day. This is because these foods improve diet quality when eaten in smaller amounts but detract from it when eaten in larger amounts. For example, whole-grain foods are a great source of low-glycemic carbohydrates, fiber, and certain vitamins and minerals, but they are also rather calorie dense, so it's best to have just a few portions of them each day.

▶ CALCULATING YOUR DAILY DQS IS SIMPLE: ASSIGN THE APPROPRIATE POINTS BASED ON HOW MANY SERVINGS OF EACH TYPE OF FOOD YOU EAT.

TABLE 2.1 DIET-QUALITY-SCORE FOOD CATEGORIES

HIGH-QUALITY FOODS	
FRUIT	Whole fresh fruits, canned and frozen fruits, and 100% fruit juices
VEGETABLES	Whole, fresh vegetables eaten cooked or raw, canned and frozen vegetables, and pureed or liquefied vegetables used in soups, sauces, and such
WHOLE GRAINS	Brown rice, amaranth, whole oats, teff, quinoa, etc., and breakfast cereals, breads, and pastas made with 100% whole grains
LEAN PROTEINS	All meats containing 10% fat or less, all seafood, and all types of nuts and seeds (including two eggs per day that count as lean proteins, too)
LOW-FAT DAIRY	Milk, cheese, yogurt, and other dairy foods made with low-fat or skim milk
ESSENTIAL FATTY ACIDS	Fish, fish oil supplements, flaxseeds, flaxseed oil supplements
LOW-QUALITY FOODS	
REFINED GRAINS	White rice, processed flours, and all breakfast cereals, pastas, breads, and other baked goods made with less than 100% whole grains
SWEETS	Candy, chocolate, pastries, desserts, soft drinks, and other sugary foods and beverages
FRIED FOODS	Snack chips, donuts, fried meats, fritters, French fries, and anything else deep fried (not including stir-fries and other foods prepared by "light" frying)
WHOLE-MILK DAIRY	Whole milk and cheeses, yogurt, ice cream, and any other dairy foods made with whole milk
FATTY PROTEINS	Any meats containing more than 10% fat

PORTIONS

What's a portion, anyway? Because the Diet Quality Score is intended to control the quality of the food you eat more than the amount, there is no need to define portions rigorously. A portion can just be an amount of food of a given type that is normal for you. For example, if you eat a sandwich for lunch most days, count the two slices of bread

TABLE 2.2 DQS SCORING BY FOOD TYPE

SERVINGS	1	2	3	4	5	6
HIGH-QUALITY FOODS						
FRUIT	2	2	2	1	0	0
VEGETABLE	2	2	2	1	0	0
LEAN PROTEIN	2	2	1	0	0	-1
WHOLE GRAIN	2	2	1	0	0	-1
LOW-FAT DAIRY	1	1	1	0	-1	-2
ESSENTIAL FATS	2	0	0	0	-1	-1
LOW-QUALITY FOODS						
REFINED GRAIN	-1	-1	-2	-2	-2	-2
SWEET	-2	-2	-2	-2	-2	-2
FRIED FOOD	-2	-2	-2	-2	-2	-2
FULL-FAT DAIRY	-1	-1	-2	-2	-2	-2
FATTY PROTEIN	-1	-1	-2	-2	-2	-2

as one serving of either whole grains or refined grains, depending on whether they are made with 100 percent whole grains or not. Just try to be consistent and honest with your portion definitions. For example, if you have a little lettuce and tomato on a sandwich, count that as half a vegetable portion, not a whole portion. If you flip out one night and eat an entire pint of ice cream, count that as two or three portions of sweets.

SCORING ANOMALIES

But wait. Shouldn't ice cream be counted as a whole-milk dairy food? There are many examples of foods that inherently belong to more than one category of the 11 total food categories in the DQS system.

There are also many foods that combine foods of more than one type. How should these be handled? Just use common sense and, again, be honest and consistent. For example, ice cream and other dairy foods with added sugar should be counted as sweets *and* as whole-milk dairy foods.

I get a lot of questions from people about how to score foods that don't fit neatly into a single box in Table 2.1. I always encourage them to make their own decisions. There's no scientifically exact way to do it, and even if there were, scientific precision wouldn't matter. The point is to score the foods in your diet accurately enough to get a reasonable assessment of your diet quality and to reliably track changes in the quality of your diet. Here are a few examples of how I score certain foods that people often ask me about:

Condiments and sauces: No score unless I eat a fairly substantial amount of a high-calorie sauce or condiment, in which case it subtracts a point from my DQS.

Energy bars: I score these as sweets if they are really just glorified candy bars. Otherwise I score them as refined grains, unless they are made primarily with whole grains, nuts, seeds, and/or real fruit, in which case I score them as whole-grain foods.

Diet soft drinks: I score these as sweets even if they have no calories because research indicates that diet soda doesn't offer any real advantage to regular soda. In terms of DQS, both qualify as poor choices.

Legumes: I count these as vegetables.

Sandwiches: Typically I score the bread as one (whole or refined) grain serving, the meat or fish as one-half to one serving of (lean or fatty) meat, the veggies as one-half to one serving of vegetables, and the cheese as one-half serving of (whole-milk or low-fat) dairy.

Soy foods: I count these as legumes, but I suggest vegetarians count them as lean proteins.

BALANCING YOUR ENERGY SOURCES

As you probably know, there are three major sources of energy, measured in calories, in the diet: carbohydrate, fat, and protein. We need all three for health and performance. Almost everyone in our society gets more than enough of each macronutrient to support general health, but an endurance athlete in the midst of strenuous training needs to take in more macronutrients than a sedentary person of the same height and weight. In fact, endurance athletes are certain to see their training suffer in one way or another if they fail to consistently get the amount of a given macronutrient needed to support optimal performance. Common symptoms of deficiency include sluggishness in workouts, slow recovery from workouts, and increased susceptibility to illness and injury. Of course, it is also possible to consume too much of one or more macronutrients. The result is the same for endurance athletes as it is for anyone else: accumulation of unwanted body fat.

During periods of race-focused training, shedding excess body fat is not a direct objective of balancing your energy sources. The direct objective is to maximize your performance in training. But maximizing your training performance will also lead to improved body composition.

The relative amounts of carbs, fats, and proteins that constitute too little and too much differ. Thus, it is important to get the right balance of macronutrients in your diet. Endurance athletes need more carbohydrate because it is a major fuel for exercise that the body is not able to store in large amounts. The more you train, the more carbohydrate you burn and thus the more you need to eat. Training increases fat and protein usage and needs, too, but not nearly as much.

Research suggests that most endurance athletes get plenty of fat and protein but not enough carbohydrate to support optimal training

▶ENDURANCE ATHLETES ARE CERTAIN TO SEE THEIR TRAINING SUFFER IF THEY FAIL TO CONSISTENTLY GET THE OPTIMAL AMOUNT OF A GIVEN MACRONUTRIENT.

performance. Endurance athletes are often advised to get 60 percent of their daily calories from carbs, but the average endurance athlete gets less than 50 percent. In reality, the 60 percent recommendation is dubious because it doesn't scale appropriately to different levels of training. In fact, athletes who train extensively generally need to get more than 60 percent of their calories from carbs, while those who train lightly need less. So it's best to ignore percentages and instead aim to get a certain absolute amount of carbohydrate in your diet appropriate to your present training volume.

Table 2.3 offers recommendations for carbohydrate intake based on training volume and goal weight. Body weight also must be considered in determining carbohydrate needs. The heavier you are, the more carbohydrate your body burns per hour of training. But it's best to base your target carbohydrate intake on your goal weight (that is, your racing weight) instead of your current weight. After all, there's no need to provide fuel for those excess fat stores that stand between you and your racing weight.

TABLE 2.3 RECOMMENDED CARBOHYDRATE INTAKE

WEEKLY TRAINING VOLUME	CARBOHYDRATE INTAKE (BASED ON GOAL WEIGHT)
≤4 HOURS	2–2.75 g/lb.
5–6 HOURS	2.75–3.25 g/lb.
7–10 HOURS	3.25–3.75 g/lb.
11–14 HOURS	3.75–4 g/lb.
15–19 HOURS	4–4.5 g/lb.
20–24 HOURS	4.5–5 g/lb.
≥25 HOURS	5–5.5 g/lb.

Once you have calculated your carbohydrate needs, it's easy to determine your fat and protein needs:

1. Multiply your daily carbohydrate target by four to determine the number of carbohydrate calories you need.

2. Subtract this number from your total daily calorie intake target. I will show you how to set that target in Chapter 4.

3. The remainder represents the number of combined fat and protein calories you need daily. About half to two-thirds of these calories should come from fat, the other one-half to one-third from protein.

These broad parameters allow for a substantial degree of individual freedom of choice in fat and protein intake. You just need to experiment until you find what works best for you. Research has proven that athletes can thrive at a variety of fat and protein intake levels, as long as the minimums are met and total caloric intake (carbohydrate, fat, and protein combined) is appropriate. In your quick start, balancing your energy stores will favor protein over carbohydrate. We will explain this fully in Chapter 3.

NUTRIENT TIMING

When you eat is as important as what you eat. A given food may affect your body differently depending on when you eat it. You must time your meals and snacks carefully to maximize your training performance and optimize your body composition. Follow these five basic rules of nutrient timing:

RULE NO. 1: EAT EARLY

If you've heard it once, you've heard it a thousand times: Breakfast is the most important meal of the day. The reason is that eating a meal shortly after waking in the morning reduces appetite throughout the remainder of the day. Thus, breakfast eaters typically eat fewer total calories over the course of the day than breakfast skippers. Breakfast eaters also tend to have higher-quality diets, perhaps because eating early reduces cravings for sweets and fatty foods. For these reasons you should try to make breakfast a routine part of your day.

RULE NO. 2: EAT OFTEN

It is better to eat three modest-size meals and two or three snacks over the course of the day than to eat just two or three very large meals, for two reasons. First, like breakfast, frequent eating keeps appetite in check and discourages overeating. Second, the body stores more food calories in body fat when large meals are consumed infrequently than when smaller meals and snacks are consumed frequently.

RULE NO. 3: EAT BEFORE EXERCISE

You will perform better and maximize the results of your workouts when your muscles and liver are well stocked with glycogen (stored carbohydrate) and when your blood glucose level is normal. This requires that you consume a meal containing at least 100 grams of carbohydrate no more than four hours before your workout. The exact size and timing of your pre-workout meals should depend on your preferences and your schedule. You may need to experiment to find the routine that works best for you. But one way or another, make it a habit to start workouts with a full fuel tank.

RULE NO. 4: EAT DURING EXERCISE

You will perform best in workouts lasting longer than one hour if you consume a carbohydrate-containing sports drink according to your thirst throughout the workout. The optimal amount of carbohydrate for performance enhancement is roughly 60 g per hour.

Some endurance athletes avoid using sports drinks during workouts for fear the calories in them (which are mostly in the form of sugar) may sabotage their efforts to shed excess body fat. This mindset is misguided.

Athletes who fast or are tempted to fast during workouts operate on the belief that the calories in ergogenic aides simply supplement the calories eaten during the rest of the day and thereby increase the day's total calorie intake. But this is not the case. Studies have shown that when athletes consume carbohydrate during exercise, they eat less during the rest of the day.[1] So by using a sports drink or energy gel

1 C. L. Melby, K. L. Osterberg, A. Resch, B. Davy, S. Johnson, and K. Davy, "Effect of Carbohydrate Ingestion during Exercise on Post-Exercise Substrate Oxidation and Energy Intake," *International Journal of Sport Nutrition and Exercise Metabolism* 12, no. 3 (September 2002): 294–309.

during workouts you get the advantage of better performance without the disadvantage of increased total daily calorie intake.

The other rationale behind restricting carbohydrate intake during workouts is the fear that less fat will be burned during the workout if you are taking in carbohydrate. This is true. Your body will burn more carbs and less fat in workouts during which you consume carbs than during workouts in which you fast. But you will actually perform better in carb-fueled workouts, and in the long run, seeking maximum performance will most benefit your body composition.

RULE NO. 5: EAT AFTER EXERCISE

After you complete a workout your body is in a special hormonal state that lasts for a couple of hours. If you eat the right nutrients while your body occupies this state, it will make much better use of the calories consumed than if you wait more than two hours to eat. Specifically, carbohydrates and proteins consumed within this window of time will be used very efficiently to replenish your muscle glycogen (i.e., muscle carbohydrate) stores and to repair and rebuild muscle tissue damaged by the workout. Taking advantage of this "metabolic recovery window" will enable you to recover faster and perform better in the next workout. It will also enhance the muscle-building and fat-burning effects of your training.

Some athletes like to consume a snack or recovery supplement immediately after completing each workout. Others wait an hour or so and then eat a full meal. Still others do both. All these options are effective. As a general rule, aim to consume roughly 0.5 g of carbohydrate per pound of bodyweight in the first few hours after exercise and approximately 1 g of protein per 4 g of carbohydrate. Be sure to drink plenty of fluids as well to rehydrate. Table 2.4 presents recommended eating schedules for athletes with various workout schedules, based on the five rules of nutrient timing.

TABLE 2.4 RACING WEIGHT SCHEDULES FOR NUTRIENT TIMING

TIME	NUTRIENT TIMING	DAILY CALORIC INTAKE	WHAT TO EAT
MORNING WORKOUT			
6:00 a.m.	Pre-workout snack		Small amount of easily absorbed high-carb drink or food (e.g., banana, sports drink)
6:15 a.m.	**WORKOUT**		Sports drink according to thirst
7:30 a.m.	**Breakfast**/post-workout recovery nutrition	20–25%	High-carb, moderate-protein, low-fat
10:00 a.m.	Midmorning snack	10%	Any high-quality foods
12:00 p.m.	**Lunch**	20–25%	Balance of high-quality foods
3:00 p.m.	Midafternoon snack	10%	Any high-quality foods
6:00 p.m.	**Dinner**	20–25%	Balance of high-quality foods
8:30 p.m.	Evening snack (optional)	5%	Any high-quality foods
NOON WORKOUT			
7:30 a.m.	**Breakfast**	20–25%	Balance of high-quality foods
10:00 a.m.	Midmorning/pre-workout snack	10%	High-carb, moderate-protein, low-fat
12:00 p.m.	**WORKOUT**		Sports drink according to thirst
1:30 p.m.	**Lunch**/post-workout nutrition	20–25%	High-carb, moderate-protein, low-fat
6:00 p.m.	**Dinner**	20–25%	Balance of high-quality foods
8:30 p.m.	Evening snack	5%	Any high-quality foods
LATE AFTERNOON WORKOUT			
7:30 a.m.	**Breakfast**	20–25%	Balance of high-quality foods
10:00 a.m.	Midmorning snack	10%	Any high-quality foods
12:00 p.m.	**Lunch**	20–25%	Balance of high-quality foods
3:00 p.m.	Midafternoon snack/ pre-workout	10%	High-carb, moderate-protein, low-fat
5:15 p.m.	**WORKOUT**		Sports drink according to thirst
7:00 p.m.	**Dinner**/post-workout nutrition	20–25%	High-carb, moderate-protein, low-fat
TWICE-A-DAY WORKOUT			
6:00 a.m.	Pre-workout snack		Small amount of easily absorbed high-carb drink or food (e.g., banana, sports drink)
6:15 a.m.	**WORKOUT**		Sports drink according to thirst
7:30 a.m.	**Breakfast**/post-workout recovery nutrition	20–25%	High-carb, moderate-protein, low-fat
10:00 a.m.	Midmorning snack	10%	Any high-quality foods
12:00 p.m.	**Lunch**	20–25%	Balance of high-quality foods
3:00 p.m.	Midafternoon snack/ pre-workout	10%	High-carb, moderate-protein, low-fat
5:15 p.m.	**WORKOUT**		Sports drink according to thirst
7:00 p.m.	**Dinner**/post-workout nutrition	20–25%	High-carb, moderate-protein, low-fat

MANAGING YOUR APPETITE

Appetite is one of the most powerful forces in human nature. When we are hungry, we eat. We are almost powerless to resist hunger's pull. This is why eating less is not a viable long-term weight-control strategy. While we cannot get lean and stay lean by overriding our appetite, however, we can do so by managing our appetite.

There are two general ways to manage appetite. First, you can eat in ways that satisfy your hunger without providing more calories than you need to support your optimal performance body weight. Maintaining a high-quality diet is one way to achieve this objective. High-quality foods are less calorically dense than low-quality foods, meaning they contain fewer calories per unit of volume. Since the volume of food has a stronger effect on satiety than the caloric content of food, by increasing your diet quality you can reduce the number of calories you consume daily without eating less and feeling hungry. Two of the nutrient-timing measures discussed in the previous section are also effective means of managing appetite: eating early and eating often.

A second way to manage your appetite is to avoid eating when you're not hungry. Research by Brian Wansink and others has shown that a substantial fraction of the calories the average person consumes each day are consumed when he or she is not physically hungry. We eat beyond our hunger when tempting foods happen to be around, when we follow habitual eating routines, when we are served or serve ourselves excessive portions and "clean our plates," and so forth.

To free yourself from the habit of eating when you're not hungry, you need do nothing more than train yourself to recognize the difference between physical hunger and mere appetite, or between "belly hunger" and "head hunger" as I like to say; eat only when you are physically hungry and only until your physical hunger is satisfied. This was shown in a recent study by researchers at the University of Firenze, Italy.[2] A group of overweight individuals was trained to

2 M. Ciampolini, D. Lovell-Smith, R. Bianchi, B. de Pont, M. Sifone, M. van Weeren, W. de Hahn, L. Borselli, and A. Pietrobelli, "Sustained Self-Regulation of Energy Intake: Initial Hunger Improves Insulin Sensitivity," *Journal of Nutrition and Metabolism*, 2010, article ID 286952 (June 2010).

recognize the signs of physical hunger (the main one being pangs in the stomach) and were instructed to eat only when they felt these sensations. Without making any other changes to their diet these individuals lost, on average, 10 pounds in five months.

TRAINING FOR RACING WEIGHT

We all know that being lean helps us perform better as endurance athletes. We also know that training helps us get leaner. But should you purposely manipulate your training system for the sake of getting leaner? In other words, if your current training practices are not sufficient to take you down to your racing weight, should you change them to burn off more fat?

Not within the training cycle. Remember, the whole point of getting leaner is to enhance race performance and not an end in itself. It's important to keep this relationship straight and always prioritize performance improvement in your training. By definition, your racing weight is the weight at which you perform best. So you can't even determine how much you should weigh on race day except by cultivating peak fitness.

If you train in the right way to maximize your performance, you will get leaner. But if you forget about performance and just focus on shedding fat, you could get leaner in ways that do not help you race any faster.

All that being said, there are some very common training errors that limit athletes' performance and prevent them from reaching their racing weight. One of these errors is failing to do enough high-intensity training. Most endurance athletes are brave enough to grind through many hours of moderate-intensity training each week, but

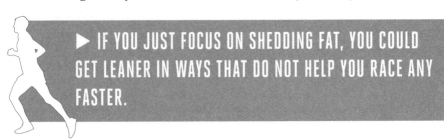

▶ IF YOU JUST FOCUS ON SHEDDING FAT, YOU COULD GET LEANER IN WAYS THAT DO NOT HELP YOU RACE ANY FASTER.

some are afraid to embrace the suffering that comes with performing high-intensity intervals that take their heart rate up to 90 to 100 percent of maximum.

That's too bad, because these types of workouts are powerful fitness builders and offer physiological benefits that no amount of moderate-intensity training can duplicate. Research shows that very high-intensity intervals have a terrific effect on body composition.[3] Every endurance athlete should make them a small but consistent part of his or her training.

Always bear in mind that the fitter you become, the faster you will go in all your workouts, including "easy" workouts. And the faster you go, the more calories you will burn in each minute of exercise and the leaner you'll get. It's a classic case of form following function.

3 M. M. Moreira, H. P. Souza, P. A. Schwingel, C. K. Sá, and C. C. Zoppi, "Effects of Aerobic and Anaerobic Exercise on Cardiac Risk Variables in Overweight Adults," *Arquivos Brasileiros de Cardiologia* 91, no. 4 (October 2008): 200–6, 219–26.

THREE

QUICK START PLAN OVERVIEW

The five key methods of body weight management for endurance athletes are improving your diet quality, balancing your energy sources, nutrient timing, managing your appetite, and training for racing weight. The first four methods are nutritional means of reducing calorie intake and body fat storage without sabotaging training performance and recovery. The fifth method entails correcting common training errors that limit both performance and improvements in body composition. The five Racing Weight methods are practiced during periods of race-focused training and also during the quick start periods that immediately precede the beginning of a new training cycle. But they must be applied differently during a quick start, whose primary objective is fast fat loss, than they are applied within the training cycle, whose primary objective is maximum race fitness. We discussed how to practice the Racing Weight methods within the training cycle in the preceding chapter. In this chapter I will explain how they are practiced differently in a quick start.

DIET QUALITY IN THE QUICK START

Although most athletes can maintain their racing weight without keeping to a perfect diet (and most people cannot sustain a perfect diet indefinitely because it's too restrictive to provide sufficient enjoyment), anyone can keep up a more or less perfect diet for a few weeks. During periods when you are trying to lose excess body fat quickly, the more you increase your diet quality, the faster you will shed excess fat. For these reasons, I recommend that you increase your diet quality from the level that normally works for you (in terms of average daily DQS) to the level of near perfection during a Racing Weight quick start.

Remember, a quick start is a four- to eight-week period preceding the beginning of formal preparation for racing, during which you try to lose weight quickly but in a way that supports your future training and racing plans. Any diet that earns a DQS of 15 or above is a fairly healthy diet, and there are many athletes able to attain their racing weight on a normal training diet that falls within the DQS range of 15–19. Such a diet can easily allow for a few unhealthy treats that keep eating sufficiently enjoyable. But within a quick start your DQS should shoot up to the 23-plus range (the maximum DQS is 29). This will require that you eliminate virtually all unhealthy foods. This isn't easy for most of us, but it's something anyone can do for four to eight weeks.

BALANCING YOUR ENERGY SOURCES IN THE QUICK START

The most important energy source, or macronutrient, within the training cycle is carbohydrate. Because carbohydrate is an important fuel for training, and serves no function other than providing energy, the more you train, the more carbohydrate you need in your diet. Getting enough carbohydrate, which most serious endurance athletes fail to do, will not only enable you to train more effectively but will also help you get leaner.

Whereas getting plenty of carbs is your main concern within the training cycle, in a quick start your carbohydrate intake should come down and your protein intake should increase to account for roughly

30 percent of your total daily calories. There are two benefits of a high-protein diet for the endurance athlete seeking to shed excess body fat prior to the start of a new training cycle. The first is that it reduces appetite, making it easier to eat less. A 2005 study from the University of Washington found that subjects voluntarily ate 14 percent less and lost weight after switching to a 30 percent protein diet.[1] This finding suggests that people can achieve the caloric deficit required for weight loss without consciously trying to reduce their eating, by simply increasing their protein intake. Other studies have shown that when people do consciously reduce their eating, they feel less hungry and thus have an easier time maintaining that caloric reduction if they also increase their protein consumption.[2]

The second benefit of a high-protein diet is that, in combination with strength training, it helps the body maintain or build muscle, so that most of the weight loss that occurs during a period of caloric restriction is in fact fat loss. Non-athletes who try to lose weight with reduced calorie intake and without exercise usually lose a fair amount of muscle mass along with body fat. This limits the desired improvements in body composition and health, and it makes weight-loss maintenance more difficult because the body's metabolic rate decreases as muscle is lost. Endurance athletes who continue to perform endurance exercise during periods of reduced calorie intake tend to lose less muscle than sedentary persons, but they still lose too much. Studies indicate that athletes who combine reduced calorie intake with strength training and high protein intake are able to preserve most or all of their muscle mass while losing as much, or even more, body fat than those who merely reduce their calories.[3]

---

1   D. S. Weigle, P. A. Breen, C. C. Matthys, H. S. Callahan, K. E. Meeuws, V. R. Burden, and J. Q. Purnell, "A High-Protein Diet Induces Sustained Reductions in Appetite, Ad Libitum Caloric Intake, and Body Weight Despite Compensatory Changes in Diurnal Plasma Leptin and Ghrelin Concentrations," *American Journal of Clinical Nutrition* 82. no. 1 (July 2005): 41–8.

2   M. Flechtner-Mors, B. O. Boehm, R. Wittmann, U. Thoma, and H. H. Ditschuneit, "Enhanced Weight Loss with Protein-Enriched Meal Replacements in Subjects with the Metabolic Syndrome," *Diabetes Metabolism Research and Reviews* 26, no. 5 (June 2010): 393–405.

3   S. Mettler, N. Mitchell, and K. D. Tipton, "Increased Protein Intake Reduces Lean Body Mass Loss During Weight Loss in Athletes," *Medicine & Science in Sports and Exercise* 42, no. 2 (February 2010): 326–37.

The average American's diet is 18 percent protein. That's already a high-protein diet when you consider that for most people a 10 percent protein diet is adequate to support optimal health. But the typical American diet still does not provide enough protein to support a maximally effective short-term weight-loss period in endurance athletes. For the best results you need to get around 30 percent protein, which requires a careful approach.

NUTRIENT TIMING IN THE QUICK START

Nutrient timing should be practiced in the same way during a quick start phase as it is within the training cycle, with one exception. During a quick start phase, some of your moderate-intensity endurance workouts should be performed in a fasted state—that is, first thing in the morning, without a preceding meal and without carbohydrate intake during the workout. This way of timing your nutrition and training to deprive your muscles of carbohydrate will force them to rely on fat and will thereby maximize the fat-burning effect of the workouts and generally enhance the fat-burning capacity of your muscles.

The downside of depriving your muscles of carbohydrate before and during long workouts is that it reduces performance. For this reason, I recommend performing mostly well-fueled workouts within the training cycle, when performance is the top priority. But in a quick start period, when rapid fat loss takes precedence, doing one prolonged fat-burning workout in a fasted state each week will help you achieve that objective.

MANAGING YOUR APPETITE IN THE QUICK START

There is a difference between eating less food and eating fewer calories. It is possible to eat fewer calories without eating less food. The best way to do that is to replace some of the calorie-dense, low-quality foods in your diet with less calorie-dense, high-quality foods.

> ▶ DURING A QUICK START PHASE, SOME OF YOUR MODERATE-INTENSITY ENDURANCE WORKOUTS SHOULD BE PERFORMED IN A FASTED STATE.

Consciously eating less is not a viable long-term weight control strategy because it produces hunger. This is why the Racing Weight system does not require athletes to eat less within race-focused training periods. However, eating less can be tolerated for short periods of time, and to lose fat quickly eating less is necessary.

Specifically, you will maintain a daily calorie deficit of a predetermined size throughout your quick start. The size and duration of this deficit should depend on how much weight you need to lose. As mentioned previously, there are three different quick start plans. Those who are 5 to 10 lbs. above their racing weight will maintain a daily deficit of 300 calories for four weeks. Those who are 11 to 20 lbs. above their racing weight will maintain a daily deficit of 400 calories for six weeks. Those who are more than 20 lbs. above their racing weight will maintain a daily deficit of 500 calories for eight weeks.

WEIGHT LOSS IN THE QUICK START

How much weight can you expect to lose on each of these quick starts? Your exact results will depend on a variety of factors, including your diet and activity level before the quick start and your genetic disposition for weight loss. As a general rule, you can expect to lose 1 pound of body weight per 3,500 calories of energy deficit you accumulate. The total energy deficit in the 300-calorie-per day, four-week quick start is 8,400 calories, which equals roughly 2.5 pounds of weight loss. The total energy deficit in the 400-calorie-per-day, six-week quick start is 16,800 calories, which equals 5 pounds of weight loss. And the total energy deficit in the eight-week, 500-calorie-deficit quick start is 28,000 calories, which equals 8 pounds of weight loss.

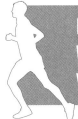

> ▶ YOU CAN EXPECT TO LOSE 1 POUND OF BODY WEIGHT PER 3,500 CALORIES OF ENERGY DEFICIT YOU ACCUMULATE.

Additional weight loss can be expected as a result of the training element of your quick start. To get an accurate estimate of this additional weight loss you would have to calculate energy expenditure in the quick start training plan you follow and compare it to energy expenditure in your current training. You would also have to account for the possible effects of the different types of training you do in the quick start—particularly high-intensity intervals and strength training—on your resting metabolism. But assuming your quick start follows an off-season break from training or a period of moderate, maintenance-level training, you can expect to lose at least 0.5 pound per week in addition to the weight you lose through your energy deficit. That brings our total estimates for *minimum* weight loss to 4.5 pounds, 8 pounds, and 12 pounds for the four-, six-, and eight-week quick starts, respectively.

It bears mentioning that all this weight loss is likely to be fat loss, whereas weight-loss plans that do not include high protein intake and the types of exercise done in a quick start typically produce muscle and water loss along with fat loss. Your body-fat measurements before and after the quick start will verify that the weight you've lost is pure body fat.

REACHING YOUR GOAL WEIGHT

As you can see, these rough weight-loss estimates fall short of the differences between current weight and racing weight that I use to match individual athletes up with a specific plan. Why are the quick starts not designed to take athletes all the way to their racing weight? Two reasons. First, it is important to avoid losing weight too quickly as an endurance athlete. An energy deficit exceeding 500 calories per day, which would be required to lose weight more quickly, would not allow you to perform well in workouts, thus sabotaging your fitness. Second, additional weight loss is almost inevitable within the race-focused training period that follows a quick start, especially if the Racing Weight system is used to guide your nutrition and training habits. So it's reasonable to anticipate additional weight loss within the training cycle.

How much additional weight can you expect to lose within a Racing Weight training cycle? Again, it depends on many factors. The Racing Weight system is designed to yield weight loss very gradually, because only very gradual weight loss supports the objective of maximizing race fitness, the primary objective within the training cycle. If you complete your quick start and begin your training cycle just 2–4 pounds above your racing weight, which is ideal, you can expect to lose that excess by the time you reach your peak training period. Athletes who begin a training cycle 10 or more pounds above their racing weight typically lose approximately 0.5 pound per week when following the Racing Weight system.

Race-focused training cycles usually last 12 to 24 weeks. So, for example, it is not unreasonable for an athlete who is 20 pounds above his racing weight to expect to lose 20 pounds and attain his racing weight in an eight-week quick start (yielding 12 pounds of weight loss), followed by a 16-week training cycle (yielding 8 additional pounds of weight loss) in which the Racing Weight system is applied.

The unfortunate reality for those who carry the most excess fat is that more than one quick start followed by a race-focused training period may be required to reach optimal racing weight. Don't let this discourage you—the positive effects of each incremental improvement on your fitness, your performance, and your overall sense of

▶ THE RACING WEIGHT SYSTEM IS DESIGNED TO YIELD WEIGHT LOSS VERY GRADUALLY, BECAUSE ONLY VERY GRADUAL WEIGHT LOSS SUPPORTS THE OBJECTIVE OF MAXIMIZING RACE FITNESS.

well-being will begin early in the quick start and push you toward your end goal. The timeline below shows how weight loss is likely to play out in both the Quick Start and throughout training. Consistency and awareness will be critical to your success.

WEIGHT LOSS AFTER THE QUICK START

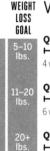

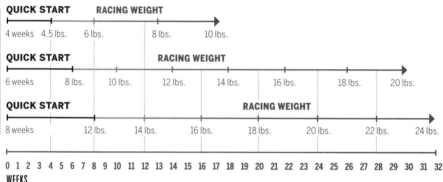

WEIGHT LOSS GOAL		
5–10 lbs.	**QUICK START** RACING WEIGHT	4 weeks 4.5 lbs. 6 lbs. 8 lbs. 10 lbs.
11–20 lbs.	**QUICK START** RACING WEIGHT	6 weeks 8 lbs. 10 lbs. 12 lbs. 14 lbs. 16 lbs. 18 lbs. 20 lbs.
20+ lbs.	**QUICK START** RACING WEIGHT	8 weeks 12 lbs. 14 lbs. 16 lbs. 18 lbs. 20 lbs. 22 lbs. 24 lbs.

0 1 2 3 4 5 6 7 8 9 10 11 12 13 14 15 16 17 18 19 20 21 22 23 24 25 26 27 28 29 30 31 32
WEEKS

WEIGHT LOSS BEYOND THE QUICK START

DON'T BE FOOLED INTO THINKING the primary goal of the Racing Weight plan is weight loss. Whereas the goal of losing weight, more specifically fat, is the main focus of the quick start, your priorities should shift as you begin a race-focused training cycle. You will continue to lose remaining excess body fat during the training cycle, but weight loss will occur more slowly as you prioritize building race fitness and fuel your body accordingly using the Racing Weight plan.

	Quick Start	Racing Weight Plan
Primary goal	Fat loss	Building race fitness
Secondary goal	Building foundational fitness	Fat loss

Furthermore, your total training duration (quick start and training cycle combined) should be determined by your race goals, not your weight loss goals. This marks another shift from the quick start, whose duration is in fact based on weight loss goals. Whether the race-focused training cycle that follows your quick start is 12 weeks, 24 weeks, or something in between is determined by the date of your chosen peak race. The closer your training cycle duration is to the maximum limit of 24 weeks, and the closer you are to your racing weight at the start of it, the more likely it is that you will attain your racing weight before your peak race.

TRAINING FOR RACING WEIGHT IN THE QUICK START

Your training during a quick start period can and should be quite different from your training within the training cycle. To start with, because the quick start precedes the beginning of race-focused training, your training volume needs to be lower. If you tried to shoulder the burden of peak training volumes before the training cycle even began, you would surely burn out before your primary race. High training volume is an effective way to stimulate fat loss, but it is not the only way. The quick start training plans I've created maximize fat loss in a volume-efficient way with a combination of very-high-intensity interval sessions, strength training, and prolonged fat-burning workouts, some of which are performed in a fasted state.

These key workouts also serve to prepare your body for the race-focused training to follow. Sessions of very short, very-high-intensity intervals burn a lot of fat, especially during the few hours after you complete them, through a phenomenon known as excess post-exercise oxygen consumption (EPOC). They also cultivate reserves of speed and power that you can develop into sustained speed in the training cycle that follows. Strength training will slightly increase your muscle mass and with it your metabolic rate, so your body burns more calories at rest. It will also give you a solid structural foundation to absorb and profit from race-focused training later. And prolonged fat-burning workouts maximize fat burning within the kind of steady endurance format needed to prepare you for the base training that will follow the quick start.

Now, you may recall that in the Introduction I described a study that seemed to show that combining high-intensity interval training with calorie restriction was less effective in increasing the

► STUDIES HAVE SHOWN THAT THE COMBINATION OF INTERVAL TRAINING AND CALORIE RESTRICTION ACTUALLY YIELDED MORE WEIGHT LOSS THAN EITHER MEASURE ALONE.

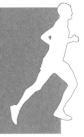

power-to-weight ratio in cyclists than either interval training or calorie restriction alone. In fact, the study showed just that. But the combination of interval training and calorie restriction actually yielded *more weight loss* than either measure alone. Since weight loss is a higher priority than performance improvement within a quick start, combining high-intensity intervals and calorie restriction in this context is appropriate. You will take full advantage of your quick start weight loss to maximize your performance later, within the training cycle.

You could map out your own quick start with these guideposts. As long as you understand how to reduce your calorie intake appropriately, how to format a sport-specific strength program, and so forth, it is unlikely that you would make any wrong turns. But if you want a guarantee of no wrong turns, I suggest you simply follow the detailed quick start meal and training plans I've devised for you.

QUICK START MEALS
AND SNACKS

The two most important characteristics of the meals and snacks you eat during a quick start are high protein content and high quality. Eating high-protein meals and snacks will satisfy your appetite with fewer calories than would normally be needed to do the job, which will enable you to maintain your desired daily calorie deficit with less hunger. It will also help you build more muscle in conjunction with your strength training, improving your body composition directly by increasing your body's muscle-to-fat ratio, and indirectly by increasing your resting metabolism so your body burns more fat at rest.

This chapter presents a selection of recommended meals and snacks that meet these two criteria. They are almost entirely made up of the food types designated as "high quality" in the Diet Quality Score system: fruits, vegetables, whole grains, lean proteins, low-fat dairy, and essential fats. They contain virtually no trace of any of the food types designated as low quality: sweets, processed grains, fatty proteins, and high-fat dairy foods. I do not believe in forcing oneself to eat "perfectly" all the time, but I do believe in trying (at least trying!) to eat perfectly during a quick start. This is the time to do everything possible to maximize your fat-loss results.

GETTING YOUR FILL OF PROTEIN

Most but not all of the meals and snacks presented here are high in protein. With them you can easily create a variety of one-day eating plans that hit the quick start protein target of 30 percent of total calories. The average American diet is 18 percent protein. While that's already a high-protein diet when you consider that for most people a 10 percent protein diet is adequate to support optimal health, the typical American diet still does not provide enough protein to support a maximally effective short-term weight-loss period in endurance athletes. Research has shown that protein intake must exceed 25 percent of total calories to have a meaningful impact on satiety,[1] and getting this much protein requires a careful approach.

Cutting down the amount of carbohydrate and fat you eat, to reduce your total calorie intake during your quick start, will itself increase the contribution of protein to the total calories in your diet. You can further increase protein as a percentage of total energy in your diet by slightly increasing the amount of healthy high-protein foods you eat. These include fish, nuts, soy foods (soybeans happen to be exactly 30 percent protein), and lean cuts of poultry and other meats.

Many athletes find it easiest to consistently hit the 30 percent mark when they include protein supplements such as protein shakes and bars in their diet. I recommend the shakes, and especially powdered protein shake mixes that contain very little else besides protein. These can be mixed into water, oatmeal, yogurt, smoothies, and other beverages and foods to increase your protein intake in a calorically

---

1 H. J. Leidy, M. Tang, C. L. Armstrong, C. B. Martin, and W. W. Campbell, "The Effects of Consuming Frequent, Higher Protein Meals on Appetite and Satiety during Weight Loss in Overweight/Obese Men," *Obesity* (Silver Spring), September 16, 2010.

efficient way. Protein bars tend to be rather calorie dense and contain a lot of highly processed artificial ingredients. Some athletes don't like the idea of consuming any protein supplements, but I consider the best protein powders to be reasonably natural and very high-quality foods, and for this reason I include them in my quick start plans. You certainly don't have to use them if you don't want to, but they are the most calorically efficient protein source (meaning they provide the most protein per calorie), so it will be a little more difficult to hit your 30 percent protein target and your calorie deficit target simultaneously without them.

KEEPING YOUR DIET SIMPLE

Your freedom of choice in food selection does not have to be limited to the meals and snacks presented in my quick start program. You should feel free to eat literally anything you want during your quick start as long as it all adds up to a roughly 30 percent protein diet, a near-maximal DQS, and the appropriate number of calories at the end of the day. With a little planning you can easily meet these standards on any sort of diet, from vegan to gluten free. The seven breakfasts, seven snacks, seven lunches, and seven dinners presented in these chapters are just suggestions that will make your quick start easier by sparing you the trouble of counting calories and protein grams and vetting quality.

Twenty-eight total meals and snacks might not seem like a ton of variety, but it's actually more variety than most of us have in our diets (how many different breakfasts have you had in the past week?), and a little monotony in the diet is actually not a bad thing when you're trying to lose fat. Studies have found that people eat more when they eat a wider variety of foods, apparently because satiety results in part from tiring of the taste of food, which obviously happens faster when you're eating just one thing.[2] And a National Weight Control

2 H. A. Raynor, R. W. Jeffrey, D. F. Tate, and R. R. Wing, "Relationship between Changes in Food Group Variety, Dietary Intake, and Weight during Obesity Treatment," *International Journal of Obesity and Related Metabolic Disorders* 28, no. 6 (June 2004): 813–20.

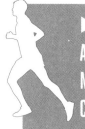

> **► DURING THE QUICK START YOUR DIET SHOULD ADD UP TO ROUGHLY 30-PERCENT PROTEIN, A NEAR-MAXIMAL DQS, AND THE APPROPRIATE NUMBER OF CALORIES AT THE END OF THE DAY.**

Registry study reported that men and women who had successfully maintained a large amount of weight loss for a long period of time had a less-varied diet than dieters who had regained lost weight.[3] The authors of this study speculated that limiting the variety of foods in the diet might help people manage their total caloric intake more effectively.

The virtue of simplicity is manifest not only in the variety of quick start meals and snacks I've selected for you but also in their preparation requirements. All the recommended quick start meals and snacks are very easy to prepare. Complete recipes are not provided, however; only basic portion size and nutrition information. If you are a confident chef, feel free to put your own twist on preparing these meals, but be sure to do so in ways that do not add a lot of extra calories. For example, try adding different spices, fresh herbs, onion, or garlic to enhance the flavor of a meal. If you need more guidance, visit food.com and enter keywords associated with any specific meal presented here in the search box to find complete recipes that use similar ingredients. In the next chapter I will show you how to put together these meals and snacks so you can hit hit your quick start daily calorie and protein targets. The ingredients listed add up to a single serving, so if your calorie needs are higher, you'll need to adjust those accordingly. To make your daily calorie computations a little easier, I present nutrition facts for 1, 1.5, and 2 servings for each meal or snack.

I've tallied the DQS for each meal and snack in order to help you become more familiar with this scoring system. Should you choose to incorporate different meals and snacks, you will want to tally your

---

3 H. A. Raynor, R. W. Jeffery, S. Phelan, J. O. Hill, and R. R. Wing, "Amount of Food Group Variety Consumed in the Diet and Long-Term Weight Loss Maintenance," *Obesity Research*, 13 (2005): 883–90.

DQS to be sure you are choosing high-quality foods. You'll notice that the DQS doesn't vary with the number of servings. This is because the DQS takes into account individually appropriate portions. For example, a petite female runner and a tall male triathlete will eat different portions of a tuna steak, amaranth, and kale dinner, but the DQS will be the same for both athletes. Be aware that the scores of some meals and snacks may vary based on what you've already eaten in the day. For example, the "Tofu with Vegetable Stir-Fry and Brown Rice" dinner is valued at 8 points on its own. But two of those points come from brown rice, a whole grain, and whole grains are worth 2 points in each of the first two servings you eat in a day, but the third serving is worth only 1 point. So if you've already eaten two whole grains when you sit down with a plate of tofu and vegetable stir fry with brown rice, it's worth 7 points instead of 8.

QUICK START BREAKFASTS

These seven breakfast menus include hot and cold, larger and smaller, and vegetarian and non-vegetarian options.

BAGEL WITH CREAM CHEESE & LOX

1 whole-wheat bagel

2 Tbsp. light cream cheese

2 tomato slices

2 oz. lox

Nutrition Facts — DQS 6

Servings	1	1.5	2
Energy	274 cal.	411 cal.	548 cal.
Carbs	31 g	46.5 g	62 g
Fat	7 g	10.5 g	14 g
Protein	19.5 g	29.3 g	39 g

BREAKFAST WRAP

1 whole-wheat tortilla (8 inches)

½ cup egg substitute*

1 cup grilled, diced green and red peppers, onions

1 oz. shredded low-fat cheddar cheese

Nutrition Facts — DQS 7

Servings	1	1.5	2
Energy	324 cal.	486 cal.	648 cal.
Carbs	28 g	42 g	56 g
Fat	11 g	16.5 g	22 g
Protein	26 g	39 g	52 g

Egg substitute is recommended instead of whole eggs because it is more protein dense and less calorie dense than whole eggs. Egg substitute is simply egg white. Feel free to use a packaged egg substitute such as Egg Beaters or use the whites of whole eggs. It's okay to use whole eggs if you much prefer their taste and/or texture.

CEREAL WITH SKIM MILK

2 cups cereal

1 cup skim milk

Nutrition Facts — DQS 3

Example: Kashi GoLean and milk

Servings	1	1.5	2
Energy	366 cal.	549 cal.	732 cal.
Carbs	72 g	108 g	144 g
Fat	2 g	3 g	4 g
Protein	34.5 g	51.8 g	69 g

MEALS

10 RECOMMENDED BREAKFAST CEREALS

SOME BREAKFAST CEREALS ARE VERY WHOLESOME, BUT OTHERS ARE CANDY IN DISGUISE. Below are some cereals that pass Racing Weight quick start standards. All are made with whole grains and do not list any form of sugar among their top two ingredients. Most are not particularly high in protein. Kashi GoLean is one of the few breakfast cereals that offers more than 30 percent of its calories from protein. There are, however, a few other cereals that, when combined with skim milk, make 30 percent protein meals. Some don't reach that protein level even with milk, but it is not necessary that every single meal you eat be 30 percent protein.

Bob's Red Mill Granola
Cheerios
Cinnamon Puffins
Ezekiel 4:9 Organic Golden Flax
Fiber One Honey Clusters
Kashi GoLean
Nature's Path Flax Plus Flakes
Post Grape-Nuts Flakes
Post Raisin Bran
Quaker Oatmeal Squares

VEGETABLE OMELET

¾ cup egg substitute
¼ cup cooked spinach (start
    with 2 cups raw)
2 Tbsp. diced tomatoes
¼ cup onions

Nutrition Facts `DQS 4`

Servings	1	1.5	2
Energy	237 cal.	356 cal.	474 cal.
Carbs	8 g	12 g	16 g
Fat	9 g	13.5 g	18 g
Protein	31 g	46.5 g	62 g

PROTEIN SMOOTHIE

1 cup low-fat yogurt
4 oz. orange juice
½ banana
1 scoop protein powder

Nutrition Facts `DQS 6`

Servings	1	1.5	2
Energy	405 cal.	607 cal.	810 cal.
Carbs	62 g	93 g	124 g
Fat	2 g	3 g	4 g
Protein	30 g	45 g	60 g

MEALS

EGG & VEGGIE SCRAMBLE

1 cup egg substitute
½ cup diced bell peppers
2 Tbsp. diced onions
¼ cup sliced mushrooms

Nutrition Facts — DQS 4

Servings	1	1.5	2
Energy	232 cal.	348 cal.	464 cal.
Carbs	8 g	12 g	16 g
Fat	8 g	12 g	16 g
Protein	32 g	48 g	64 g

PROTEIN TEFF PORRIDGE

1 cup teff
1 scoop protein powder
¾ cup date pieces
½ cup walnut pieces
1 Tbsp. butter
¼ cup skim milk

Nutrition Facts — DQS 8

Servings	1	1.5	2
Energy	381 cal.	572 cal.	762 cal.
Carbs	56 g	84 g	112 g
Fat	7 g	10.5 g	14 g
Protein	30 g	45 g	60 g

QUICK START SNACKS

You won't find potato chips on this list of healthy snacks!

CELERY STICKS WITH PEANUT BUTTER

8 celery sticks
2 Tbsp. reduced-fat old-fashioned
  peanut butter

Nutrition Facts — DQS 1

Servings	1	1.5	2
Energy	208 cal.	312 cal.	416 cal.
Carbs	8 g	12 g	16 g
Fat	16 g	24 g	32 g
Protein	8 g	12 g	16 g

ENERGY BAR

Nutrition Facts · DQS 2

Example: Forze Bar

Servings	1	1.5	2
Energy	160 cal.	240 cal.	320 cal.
Carbs	22 g	33 g	44 g
Fat	8 g	12 g	16 g
Protein	8 g	12 g	16 g

Only real-food energy bars made with fruit, whole grains, nuts, etc. and with minimal added sugar are acceptable in a Racing Weight quick start. Examples are Forze Bar, Greens+ Natural Energy Bar, Perfect Foods Bar, and PowerBar Nut Naturals Bar.

FRUIT SMOOTHIE WITH PROTEIN

8 oz. orange juice

1 fresh banana

½ cup frozen strawberries

½ cup frozen blueberries

1 scoop whey protein powder

Nutrition Facts · DQS 6

Servings	1	1.5	2
Energy	417 cal.	626 cal.	834 cal.
Carbs	72 g	108 g	144 g
Fat	2 g	3 g	4 g
Protein	20 g	30 g	40 g

AVOIDING HIDDEN SUGAR

ALMOST ALL FLAVORED YOGURTS CONTAIN ADDED SUGAR. A little sugar in your yogurt won't kill you, but it's so unnecessary. Plain yogurt already contains lactose sugar and fruit sweetens it plenty. That's why I recommend you buy plain yogurt and add your own fruit to sweeten it.

Almost all packaged sandwich breads also contain sugar, as with yogurt. I don't know why, because it's just not needed. Shop at health food stores instead of supermarkets to find the few brands of bread out there without some type of sugar on the ingredients list.

Save the added sugar for foods that really "need" it, like that little square of dark chocolate you might allow yourself after dinner!

MEALS

JERKY

1 oz. jerky (beef, turkey, fish, or
    venison)

Nutrition Facts   DQS 2

Example: turkey jerky

Servings	1	1.5	2
Energy	69 cal.	104 cal.	138 cal.
Carbs	0 g	0 g	0 g
Fat	0.5 g	0.8 g	1 g
Protein	13 g	19.5 g	26 g

YOGURT WITH FRUIT

1 cup plain low-fat yogurt
¼ cup fruit (peach, blueberries, etc.)
1 Tbsp. 100% fruit preserves*
    (peach, blueberry, etc.)

Nutrition Facts   DQS 3

Example: blueberries and blueberry preserves

Servings	1	1.5	2
Energy	176 cal.	264 cal.	352 cal.
Carbs	33 g	44 g	66 g
Fat	0 g	0 g	0 g
Protein	11 g	16.5 g	22 g

100% fruit means fruit is the only ingredient on the label.

PROTEIN SHAKE

PICK YOUR PROTEIN: SOY OR WHEY. The best-quality protein shake mixes are to be found at your local natural foods market (e.g., Whole Foods). An increasing number of regular supermarkets also carry a small selection of these products.

SOY PROTEIN SHAKE

1 scoop soy protein shake mix
8 oz. skim milk

Nutrition Facts   DQS 3

Example: Genisoy Vanilla Shake

Servings	1	1.5	2
Energy	220 cal.	330 cal.	440 cal.
Carbs	28 g	42 g	56 g
Fat	1 g	1.5 g	2 g
Protein	24 g	36 g	48 g

WHEY PROTEIN SHAKE

1 scoop whey protein shake powder

8 oz. water or skim milk

Nutrition Facts   `DQS 2`

Example: Designer Whey Vanilla Protein Shake with water

Servings	1	1.5	2
Energy	100 cal.	150 cal.	200 cal.
Carbs	3 g	4.5 g	6 g
Fat	2 g	3 g	4 g
Protein	18 g	27 g	36 g

Nutrition Facts

Nutritional facts for shake with skim milk:

Servings	1	1.5	2
Energy	186 cal.	279 cal.	372 cal.
Carbs	15 g	22.5 g	30 g
Fat	2.4 g	3.6 g	4.8 g
Protein	26.5 g	39.8 g	53 g

WHOLE FRUIT

1 whole apple, banana, orange, pear, etc.

Nutrition Facts   `DQS 2`

Example: one apple

Servings	1	1.5	2
Energy	116 cal.	174 cal.	232 cal.
Carbs	31 g	46.5 g	62 g
Fat	0 g	0 g	0 g
Protein	1 g	1.5 g	2 g

MEALS

BEYOND WHOLE WHEAT

QUICK: NAME FOUR WHOLE GRAINS. Let's see, there's whole wheat, brown rice, oats and . . . what else? Don't feel bad. Even the most health-conscious eaters often stick to the same three foods as their whole-grain sources. But there are lots of other options with different tastes and nutrient profiles to give your palate and your body some welcome variety. Following are five alternative whole grains to try. Most can be found at your local natural foods market.

AMARANTH: These seeds have a creamy consistency when cooked and an earthy taste. Amaranth is among the most fiber-rich and protein-rich grains.

BUCKWHEAT: Also called kasha, buckwheat has a strong, distinctive taste and is rich in the phytonutrient rutin.

QUINOA: This grain provides one of the broadest amino acid spectrums in the plant kingdom and is appreciated for its nutty taste.

SPELT: Similar to wheat, spelt contains more protein, fiber, magnesium, selenium, and niacin than its close grain cousin. It has a chewy consistency when cooked and a light sweetness on the tongue.

TEFF: This grain cooks into a porridge-like consistency and has a slightly malty taste. It's a great source of iron, calcium, fiber, and B vitamins, among other nutrients.

QUICK START LUNCHES

You can't go wrong by including any of these lunch menus in your quick start.

TURKEY SANDWICH

2 slices high-protein bread
   (e.g., P28 bread)
3 oz. lean turkey breast
1 Tbsp. mustard
Onion, lettuce, tomato

Nutrition Facts   DOS 5

Servings	1	1.5	2
Energy	342 cal.	513 cal.	684 cal.
Carbs	21 g	31.5 g	42 g
Fat	10 g	15 g	20 g
Protein	42 g	63 g	84 g

CHICKEN, BEAN & VEGGIE BURRITO

1 whole-wheat tortilla (8 inches)
3 oz. shredded grilled chicken
¼ cup black beans
½ cup grilled red and green bell
    peppers, onions
3 Tbsp. avocado, pureed
2 Tbsp. salsa

Nutrition Facts `DQS 6`

Example: one well-filled eight-inch tortilla

Servings	1	1.5	2
Energy	485 cal.	728 cal.	970 cal.
Carbs	54 g	81 g	108 g
Fat	13.5 g	20.3 g	27 g
Protein	40 g	60 g	80 g

CHICKEN CAESAR SALAD

2 cups romaine lettuce
2 Tbsp. low-calorie Caesar salad
    dressing
3 oz. chicken breast

Nutrition Facts `DQS 4`

Servings	1	1.5	2
Energy	186 cal.	279 cal.	372 cal.
Carbs	13 g	19.5 g	26 g
Fat	2 g	3 g	4 g
Protein	29 g	43.5 g	58 g

Nutrition Facts

For two wraps:

Servings	1	1.5	2
Energy	390 cal.	585 cal.	780 cal.
Carbs	45 g	67.5 g	90 g
Fat	6 g	9 g	12 g
Protein	37 g	55.5 g	74 g

To eat as wraps, add 2 whole-wheat tortillas.

TUNA MELT

1 slice whole-wheat bread
2 oz. albacore tuna
1 Tbsp. mayonnaise
Diced onions to taste
Tomato slice
1 deli slice provolone cheese

Nutrition Facts `DQS 4.5`

Servings	1	1.5	2
Energy	281 cal.	422 cal.	562 cal.
Carbs	24 g	36 g	48 g
Fat	9 g	13.5 g	18 g
Protein	26 g	39 g	52 g

MEALS

STEAK WRAP

1 9-inch whole-wheat tortilla
3 oz. London broil steak strips
1 cup grilled red & green peppers,
    onion
2 Tbsp. reduced-fat Russian salad
    dressing

Nutrition Facts · DQS 6

Servings	1	1.5	2
Energy	356 cal.	534 cal.	712 cal.
Carbs	47 g	70.5 g	94 g
Fat	7.5 g	11.3 g	15 g
Protein	25 g	37.5 g	50 g

LENTIL & SAUSAGE SOUP

12 oz. lentil soup
2 oz. sliced lean kielbasa

Nutrition Facts · DQS 4

Servings	1	1.5	2
Energy	320 cal.	480 cal.	640 cal.
Carbs	51 g	76.5 g	102 g
Fat	5.5 g	8.3 g	11 g
Protein	19.5 g	29.3 g	39 g

PEANUT BUTTER & JELLY SANDWICH

2 slices protein bread
2 Tbsp. old-fashioned reduced-fat
    peanut butter
1 Tbsp. 100% strawberry preserves

Nutrition Facts · DQS 2

For one sandwich:

Servings	1	1.5	2
Energy	510 cal.	765 cal.	1,020 cal.
Carbs	40 g	60 g	80 g
Fat	23 g	34.5 g	46 g
Protein	36 g	54 g	72 g

Don't laugh—no less an endurance athlete than six-time Hawaii Ironman world champion Dave Scott eats a PB&J sandwich almost every day. Use these "grown-up" ingredients and you'll enjoy a sandwich that is tastier and healthier than the ones you found in your school lunchbox.

GUIDELINES FOR VEGETARIANS AND VEGANS

IF YOU ARE A VEGETARIAN OR VEGAN, you have probably noticed that only a fraction of the meals and snacks presented here are appropriate for you. Don't fret. There are plenty of things you can eat for breakfast, lunch, dinner, and snacks that will collectively meet your quick start standards, including the 30 percent protein standard that is, admittedly, a little tougher for vegetarians and vegans to meet. Here are some suggestions:

For breakfast, rely on high-protein cereals such as Kashi GoLean and pour soy, hemp, rice, coconut, or almond milk over them if you are vegan, or skim cow's milk if you consume it. Naturally, lacto-ovo vegetarians may also eat any of the egg-based breakfasts presented in this chapter, while vegans can transform any grain-based breakfast (old-fashioned oatmeal, teff porridge, buckwheat pancakes, etc.) into a high-protein repast by mixing in a plant-based protein powder.

Speaking of plant-based protein powders, if you are a vegan you will almost certainly need to rely on one or more such products daily to meet your elevated quick start protein requirement. In addition to soy protein powder, hemp, rice, and pea protein powders are available.

There is a variety of plant food products besides protein powders that can help you bootstrap your way to high-protein intake, including other soy products such as tofu, tempeh, soy yogurt, and edamame; seitan, or wheat gluten, which is used to make veggie burgers and such; and protein-fortified breads such as hemp bread.

As a vegetarian, you would do well to emphasize bean-based soups, stews, chilis, and other dishes in your quick start dinners. You are probably aware that legumes such as lentils (30 percent protein exactly) are the most protein-rich plant foods. But there are many plant foods that get a high percentage of their calories from protein even though they don't contain large absolute amounts of protein (or calories in general). To name a few:

Asparagus	34%
Broccoli	27%
Mushrooms	43%
Spinach	39%

(Of course, mushrooms are technically a fungus, not a plant food.)

By packing your quick start diet with these foods, you can eat very normally and still meet your protein requirement. You'll have to eat a lot of asparagus and such to get enough calories in the day, but that's not such a bad thing, and it's also life as a vegetarian or vegan athlete.

MEALS

QUICK START DINNERS

All seven of these dinners have the high protein content and low calorie density you're looking for in quick start meals.

SALMON, BROWN RICE & SNOW PEAS

½ broiled salmon fillet

⅔ cup brown rice

½ cup steamed snow peas

Nutrition Facts · DQS 6

Servings	1	1.5	2
Energy	480 cal.	720 cal.	960 cal.
Carbs	33 g	49.5 g	66 g
Fat	15 g	22.5 g	30 g
Protein	43 g	64.5 g	86 g

CHICKEN & BROCCOLI STIR-FRY

⅔ cup broccoli crowns

4 oz. chicken tenders

½ cup brown rice

2 Tbsp. low-sodium soy sauce

Nutrition Facts · DQS 6

Servings	1	1.5	2
Energy	249 cal.	374 cal.	498 cal.
Carbs	29 g	43.5 g	58 g
Fat	2 g	3 g	4 g
Protein	28 g	42 g	56 g

TOFU & VEGETABLE STIR-FRY

¼ cup baby corn

¼ cup sliced bell peppers

¼ cup sliced mushrooms

¼ cup cooked bok choy (use 2 cups fresh)

4 oz. tofu cubes

½ cup brown rice

2 Tbsp. low-sodium soy sauce

Nutrition Facts · DQS 8

Servings	1	1.5	2
Energy	271 cal.	407 cal.	542 cal.
Carbs	35 g	52.5 g	70 g
Fat	6 g	9 g	12 g
Protein	18 g	27 g	36 g

LEAN PROTEINS

PROTEIN IS ALWAYS IMPORTANT, but it's especially important during a quick start, when you aim to get 30 percent of your daily calories from protein to control appetite and preserve muscle mass. Not all protein sources are equal, though. Some high-protein foods are also high-fat foods. You'll want to avoid these for the most part during your quick start, not because you're at any risk of eating too much fat, but because you're trying to limit calories, and fat has more than twice as many calories per gram as protein and carbohydrate. What you want instead are low-fat, lean proteins. Here's a list of recommended lean protein sources with protein and fat contents per serving:

Lean Protein Sources	Protein	Fat
Baked beans	12 g	1 g
Chicken breast	27 g	3 g
Egg substitute	15 g	4 g
Fish, wild caught (e.g., Atlantic cod)*	19 g	1 g
Ground beef (95% lean)	18 g	3 g
Lentils	9 g	0.5 g
London broil	30 g	5 g
Pork tenderloin	22 g	3 g
Tofu	10 g	6 g
Tuna, canned (water packed)	21 g	3 g
Turkey breast	24 g	1 g
Whey protein powder	18 g	2 g
Yogurt (low fat)	13 g	4 g

Note that the manner of preparing meats and fish also affects how lean they are. Baking, roasting, broiling, grilling, and roasting generally add little or no fat calories to meats and fish, while frying does.

* Protein and fat contents in fish vary by species.

TURKEY BREAST, QUINOA & BRUSSELS SPROUTS

6 oz. roasted turkey breast

½ cup quinoa

1 cup boiled Brussels sprouts

Nutrition Facts · DQS 6

Servings	1	1.5	2
Energy	550 cal.	825 cal.	1,100 cal.
Carbs	65 g	97.5 g	130 g
Fat	7 g	10.5 g	14 g
Protein	55 g	82.5 g	110 g

MEALS

PORK TENDERLOINS, SWEET POTATO & SWISS CHARD

4 oz. roasted pork tenderloins
4 oz. roasted sweet potatoes
1 cup boiled Swiss chard

Nutrition Facts			DQS 6
Servings	1	1.5	2
Energy	382 cal.	573 cal.	764 cal.
Carbs	40 g	60 g	80 g
Fat	12 g	18 g	24 g
Protein	26 g	39 g	52 g

TUNA STEAK, AMARANTH & KALE

8 oz. tuna steak
¼ cup amaranth seeds
1 cup boiled kale

Nutrition Facts			DQS 6
Servings	1	1.5	2
Energy	587 cal.	881 cal.	1,174 cal.
Carbs	41 g	61.5 g	82 g
Fat	22 g	33 g	44 g
Protein	59 g	88.5 g	118 g

TURKEY MEATLOAF, BLACK BEAN & CORN SALAD

6 oz. meatloaf made with lean
    ground turkey
½ cup black bean and corn salad

Nutrition Facts			DQS 4
Servings	1	1.5	2
Energy	444 cal.	666 cal.	888 cal.
Carbs	35 g	52.5 g	70 g
Fat	16 g	18 g	32 g
Protein	37 g	55.5 g	74 g

AND TO DRINK

You probably noticed that there are no beverages included in these meals. Obviously, you will want to drink something with most of your meals and snacks, as well as throughout the day, to satisfy your thirst and stay hydrated. Here are some guidelines for beverages during the Racing Weight quick start:

- Drink as much water as you want, and try to have water handy throughout the day so you are easily able to drink whenever you are thirsty.
- As much as possible, avoid beverages that subtract from your Diet Quality Score. You get one freebie each day.

- Drink as much 100 percent fruit juice as you like, but be aware that it adds a lot of calories to your diet without much of a satiating effect and is very low in protein.
- Drink up to three cups of coffee or green tea per day, if that's your habit and you tolerate caffeine well, but sweeten it little or not at all.

For a better idea of how some drinks dilute your DQS, see Table 4.1. You will notice that all beverages containing added sugar, all beverages containing fat, and all alcoholic beverages will negatively affect your DQS. Yes, this also includes all beverages containing artificial sweeteners because these drinks are associated with weight gain even though they contain no calories.

You should also be aware of what constitutes a serving. A bottled soft drink is likely 1.5 or 2 servings. A pint of beer is more than one serving. You get the picture.

TABLE 4.1 DQS SCORING OF DRINKS

SERVINGS	1	2	3	4+
HIGH-QUALITY DRINKS				
PROTEIN SHAKES (low fat, low carb)	2	Count as lean proteins		
SKIM MILK	1	Count as low-fat dairy		
SPORTS DRINKS (during exercise)	0	0	0	0
WATER	0	0	0	0
COFFEE & TEA (unsweetened/lightly sweetened)	0	0	0	–1
LOW-QUALITY DRINKS				
ALCOHOL (beer, wine, spirits)	0	–2	–2	–2
COFFEE & TEA (sweetened, cappuccino, latte, chai)	–2	–2	–2	–2
ENERGY DRINKS (Red Bull, Monster, etc.)	–2	–2	–2	–2
PROTEIN SHAKES (high fat or high carb)	–2	–2	–2	–2
SOFT DRINKS	–2	–2	–2	–2
WHOLE MILK	–2	–2	–2	–2

There are countless other meals and snacks that would fit into a quick start plan, provided they meet the requirements of being high-quality foods that are also high in protein. It's my hope that by using these options you can spend less time in the kitchen and avoid the hassle of calculating nutritional facts, leaving you more time and energy for training.

QUICK START
MEAL PLANS

t is not always easy to eat a predetermined number of calories every day. Nor is it necessary at most times. But when you are trying to achieve fast weight loss in a Racing Weight quick start, it is important to eat a targeted number of calories each day throughout the phase's four- to eight-week duration. In a quick start you need to create a moderate-size calorie deficit large enough to promote fat loss but not so large that it sabotages your training. Calculating an appropriate daily calorie target and counting calories daily throughout the quick start will ensure that you achieve this balance and get the results you seek. While it requires some effort, this effort is only required for four to eight weeks. That's something all of us can do. And if you use the meal plans presented in this chapter, you don't really have to count calories because the plans will do it for you.

To determine your quick start daily calorie target, you need to determine how many calories your body burns daily and how many pounds you need to lose to be at your racing weight. You learned how to estimate your racing weight in Chapter 1. If you have not yet gotten the body-fat percentage measurement you need to generate that estimate, be sure to do it before you begin your quick start. When that's done, subtract your racing weight from your current weight to find your weight loss goal and suggested daily calorie deficit.

CALCULATING CALORIES

Now it's time to calculate how many calories your body burns every day.

STEP 1: CALCULATE CALORIES BURNED DURING EXERCISE

Start by using an online activity calculator (racingweight.com) to calculate how many calories you burn in training in a typical day.

If the amount of exercise you do varies from day to day throughout the week, then use a daily average for the week for your calculations. If you plan to closely follow one of the training plans in Chapters 7, 8, or 9, then use that particular workout schedule for your calculations. Total up the number of calories you will burn in the first week of workouts in your chosen plan and divide that number by seven to get a daily average. You will also need to note the average number of hours you spend training each day. This will factor into your calculation in Step 3. Don't worry about the fact that you will burn significantly more calories on some days than others. It's the average that matters. While some sports nutritionists advise athletes to attempt to increase and reduce their calorie intake in proportion to daily flux in their calorie expenditure, I think this effort is more trouble than it's worth. There's no evidence that maintaining a consistent calorie deficit every day, despite fluctuations in energy expenditure, yields better results than eating a consistent number of calories every day. And the latter is certainly much easier.

The training load increases gradually from week to week in the quick start training plans. Does this mean you should recalculate your daily calorie target each week? You could, but it's not necessary, as the change is small. For example, in the final week of an eight-week high-volume quick start training plan you will burn roughly 50 calories a day more through exercise than in week one. And this assumes no change in weight. Factoring in weight loss, there will be virtually no difference in the amount of energy you burn in training from week to week in the quick start.

STEP 2: CALCULATE CALORIES BURNED DURING SLEEP

You've probably heard of basal metabolic rate (BMR), which is the number of calories your body burns at rest over 24 hours. To determine the number of calories you use daily outside of exercise, it is necessary to first calculate your BMR. Here are the standard BMR formulas for men and women:

English BMR Formula

Women: BMR = 655 + (4.35 x weight in pounds) + (4.7 x height in inches) – (4.7 x age in years)

Men: BMR = 66 + (6.23 x weight in pounds) + (12.7 x height in inches) – (6.8 x age in years)

Metric BMR Formula

Women: BMR = 655 + (9.6 x weight in kilos) + (1.8 x height in cm) – (4.7 x age in years)

Men: BMR = 66 + (13.7 x weight in kilos) + (5 x height in cm) – (6.8 x age in years)

Now take your BMR and divide it by 24 to find the calories burned during every hour of sleep (your baseline BMR). Finally, multiply this number by the average number of hours you sleep each night.

STEP 3: CALCULATE CALORIES BURNED THROUGH NON-EXERCISE ACTIVITY

Note that BMR does not include extra calories burned in any activity, including non-exercise activities such as working at a desk. So to get a good estimate of how many calories you use daily outside of exercise, you must modify the hourly BMR estimate you get from the above formulas to account for activities of daily living.

The average person with a non-physical job burns about 15 percent of his or her BMR per day through non-exercise activity. Most endurance athletes would fall into this category. Your day might involve more activity outside of training, such as a light hike with the dog or a brisk daily walk, or perhaps your profession is more active. Select the appropriate multiplier from the chart below:

ACTIVITY LEVEL	MULTIPLY BMR BY
Non-physical job & lifestyle	1.15
Non-physical job & somewhat active lifestyle	1.2
Physical job	1.3

Multiply your baseline BMR by this number. Now take the hours remaining in your day (whatever is left after exercising and sleeping) and multiply that number by your adjusted hourly BMR. This is the average number of calories you use daily outside of exercise.

STEP 4: CALCULATE TOTAL CALORIES BURNED DAILY

By now your have all of the numbers you need. The sum of the three calculations in Steps 1, 2, and 3 is your daily calories burned.

APPLYING YOUR CALORIE DEFICIT

Of course, the number of calories your body burns daily is also the number of calories you would need to eat daily to maintain your current body weight. Thus, determining how many calories you will eat each day during your quick start is as easy as subtracting your target deficit from your daily calorie expenditure. For example, if your calculations reveal that your body uses approximately (and these numbers are approximate) 2,850 calories per day, and you hope to lose 11 to 20 pounds, you will apply a deficit of 400 calories, and you will aim to eat 2,450 calories per day (2,850 − 400). You could use the 2,500-calorie meal plan found at the end of this chapter as a basis for your quick start plan.

GOAL FOR WEIGHT LOSS	CALORIE DEFICIT
5–10 lbs.	300
11–20 lbs.	400
20+ lbs.	500

HITTING THE TARGET

It is not necessary to consume exactly your target number of calories every day throughout an entire quick start to get the results you seek. In fact, it is not even possible. Calorie counting is an inexact science. The only way to precisely determine the number of calories you consume would be to have an exact duplicate of every meal and snack you eat combusted in a calorimeter, which is the device used to measure the caloric content of foods. The word "impractical" does not even begin to describe the trouble and expense of such a commitment. Fortunately, the word "unnecessary" describes it quite well. You can be confident of achieving the results you seek in your quick start by making a merely reasonable and consistent effort to hit your daily calorie target. Here are some guidelines for that effort.

Plan ahead.

If you wake up each morning having little idea what you will eat, you will find it difficult to hit your daily calorie target. Going by feel and hoping the foods you select over the course of the day add up to the desired total number of calories is not a winning strategy.

You will be much better off planning each day's eating in advance so you know it adds up. At the very least, keep a running total of the calories in the foods you eat throughout the day so you can make appropriate choices for the remaining meals and snacks of the day as you go along.

Eat the recommended meals and snacks.

Relying on the recommended quick start meals and snacks presented in the previous chapter will help you hit your daily calorie target in two ways. First, you know how many calories are in each, so you can easily use them to create one-day eating plans that deliver the right total number of calories. Second, most of these meals and snacks have low calorie densities, so the calories will tend to add up more slowly over the course of the day when you rely on them than will be the case when you eat other foods.

Also, keep in mind that your daily calorie target is not the only nutritional target you need to hit in your quick start. You also need to get roughly 30 percent of your calories from protein. Most of the recommended meals and snacks are high in protein; thus, you'll have an easier time meeting your quick start protein requirement with them.

Read labels and use online nutrition information resources.

There's no reason you cannot rely on the recommended meals and snacks exclusively in your quick start. But there's also no reason you cannot include any number of other meals and snacks. If you do stray from the list, you'll need to gather nutritional information for those other meals and snacks and use it to ensure that you hit your calorie and protein targets. Read nutrition labels on those foods that have them, get nutritional information sheets from the restaurants where you dine, and use online resources such as food.com to get calorie, carbohydrate, fat, and protein counts for non-labeled foods you eat (such as fruits and vegetables).

Manipulate portion sizes.

The calorie counts in the recommended meals and snacks are specific to the given portion sizes. These portion sizes may or may not be appropriate for you. For example, suppose you were to randomly choose one recommended breakfast, one lunch, one dinner, and two snacks from the offerings in the preceding chapter. It is unlikely that the total number of calories in this one-day food plan would match your target. One way to get it closer, whether that means adding or subtracting calories, is to fiddle with the portion sizes. Let's say your randomly chosen menu includes a breakfast of cereal and milk, and that the total number of calories in that menu leaves you 183 calories short of your target. There are 366 calories in the suggested serving size for cereal and milk. So one way to make up the deficit would be to increase your portion of cereal and milk by half—that is, to eat three cups of cereal with 1.5 cups of skim milk, instead of two cups of cereal with one cup of milk.

You may also increase or decrease portion sizes of individual items in meals containing more than one item, but this is a bit trickier because the meals give only calorie amounts per meal and do not provide calorie amounts per individual item. So, for example, if you want to increase the number of calories you get from the recommended dinner of broiled salmon, brown rice, and steamed snow peas by increasing the size of the salmon portion, you'll need to look up the calorie content of salmon on food.com or elsewhere to make the right adjustment.

Add extras and side items.

Another simple way to add calories to the day's total you get from a selection of recommended meals and snacks is to add extras and side items. I deliberately excluded beverages from all the recommended meals and also excluded commonly eaten side items from the recommended lunches to make it easy to add calories in this way. Thus, you can add 110 calories (and two grams of protein) to your breakfast by adding an eight-ounce glass of orange juice, add

212 calories to your lunch by adding a bag of whole-grain SunChips and an apple, and so forth.

Manipulate your eating frequency.

A third, very easy way to adjust the total number of calories you get in a one-day selection of recommended meals and snacks is to manipulate your eating frequency, and specifically the number of snacks you eat. If your daily calorie target is quite low, you may choose to eat no snacks—just breakfast, lunch, and dinner. If your daily calorie target is relatively high, you may choose to eat as many as three snacks: a midmorning snack between breakfast and lunch, a midafternoon snack between lunch and dinner, and an evening snack after dinner.

Note that the recommended snacks are relatively low in calories, so this method is not the way to achieve a major increase in your daily calorie totals, although you can add a significant number of calories to your day by planning multiple-item snacks (e.g., a protein shake and a peach as a midafternoon snack). Also, because the recommended snacks are low in calories, you can eat two or three snacks a day even if your daily calorie target is low. For example, you could eat baby carrots with light ranch dressing midmorning and dried fruit midafternoon and increase your total energy supply for the day by a scant 214 calories. So if your daily calorie target is low and you cannot keep your appetite in check with breakfast, lunch, and dinner only, go ahead and snack.

Develop a routine.

The more routine you bring to your daily eating patterns, the less mental work you will have to do to hit your daily calorie and protein targets. In the most extreme case, you could choose a breakfast, lunch, dinner, and one or more snacks that provide your energy and protein allotments and eat them every day for the full duration of your quick start. I don't really recommend that, but at the same time I encourage you to eat as repetitively as you please in your quick start for the sake of making calorie and protein control easy. As I explained in Chapter 4, repetition in the diet is not the evil it is often made out to be, and it's helpful to those trying to control their caloric intake and lose excess body fat.

Use protein shakes to make up protein "deficits."

The sample quick start meal plans presented in the next section meet specific calorie targets and also meet the quick start's 30 percent protein requirement. I must confess that it took some work on my part to develop plans that satisfied calorie and protein standards simultaneously. Creating a meal plan that provides a certain number of calories is easy. Creating a meal plan that contains a certain amount of protein is also easy. Creating a meal plan that provides a certain number of calories *and* contains a certain amount of protein is more challenging. You'll see for yourself if you choose to create your own meal plans in your quick start.

The easiest way to surmount this challenge is to focus on your calorie target in planning your eating and to use protein shakes to make up any deficits in protein. Protein shakes—at least the ones I recommend—are almost pure protein, so they allow for a lot of flexibility in adjusting your daily protein intake.

For example, suppose your daily calorie target is 2,000. Thirty percent of 2,000 calories is 600 calories. So your daily protein calorie target is 600. Since most nutrition labels list protein contents in grams rather than calories, it's easier to aim for a protein grams target than a protein calories target. There are four calories per gram of protein. So if your protein calories target is 600, your protein grams target is 150. Let's say you plan a day's eating that provides 2,000 calories and only 114 grams of protein. You can make up your 36-gram protein deficit in one fell swoop by consuming two servings of the protein shake given as an example in the previous chapter. (That's not to say that you would want to habitually drink two protein shakes to reach your daily requirement, but in a pinch it's an easy solution.)

There's only one small problem: Those two servings will provide 200 calories in addition to 36 grams of protein, increasing your day's calorie total to 2,200. So you'll also need to subtract 200 non-protein calories from your meal plan. If you can't get the numbers to work out exactly, don't sweat it. Again, a reasonable and consistent effort to hit your quick start calorie and protein targets is enough to produce the results you seek.

You can use the breakdown in Table 5.1 to quickly estimate your individual protein requirements based on your daily calorie intake.

TABLE 5.1 HITTING YOUR DAILY
PROTEIN TARGET IN THE QUICK START

TOTAL CALORIES	PROTEIN CALORIES	TOTAL PROTEIN (G)
1,500	450	112.5
1,600	480	120.0
1,700	510	127.5
1,800	540	135.1
1,900	570	142.5
2,000	600	150.0
2,100	630	157.5
2,200	660	165.0
2,300	690	172.5
2,400	720	180.0
2,500	750	187.5
2,600	780	195.0
2,700	810	202.5
2,800	840	210.0
2,900	870	217.5
3,000	900	225.0
3,100	930	232.5
3,200	960	240.0
3,300	990	247.5
3,400	1,020	255.0
3,500	1,050	262.5

SAMPLE QUICK START MEAL PLANS

Following are three sample one-week quick start meal plans, with daily energy targets of 1,500 calories, 2,000 calories, 2,500 calories, and 3,000 calories, plus a one-day sample vegetarian quick start meal plan.

1,500 CALORIES PER DAY			
DAY	DIET	TOTAL CALORIES	PROTEIN CALORIES
MON.	Bagel with cream cheese & lox; orange juice Chicken, bean & veggie burrito Low-fat yogurt with fruit Salmon, brown rice & snow peas	1,525	464 (30%)
TUE.	Breakfast wrap; plum Tuna melt (2 servings) Soy protein shake Tofu & vegetable stir-fry Grapes (1 cup)	1,497	480 (31%)
WED.	Cereal with skim milk with ½ sliced banana; orange juice Turkey jerky Steak wrap; spinach salad Turkey breast, quinoa & Brussels sprouts Peach	1,501	492 (33%)
THU.	Vegetable omelet; orange juice Whey protein shake Turkey sandwich; SunChips; apple Pork tenderloins, sweet potato & Swiss chard Strawberries	1,482	446 (30%)

Continued on next page

1,500 Calories per Day, *continued*

DAY	DIET	TOTAL CALORIES	PROTEIN CALORIES
FRI.	Protein smoothie Celery sticks with peanut butter Chicken Caesar salad Tuna steak, amaranth & kale Pear	1,507	504 (33%)
SAT.	Egg & veggie scramble; orange juice Low-fat yogurt with fruit Lentil & sausage soup; toasted protein bread with blueberry spreadable fruit Energy bar Chicken & broccoli stir-fry; glass white wine Peach	1,521	458 (30%)
SUN.	Protein teff porridge; orange juice Chicken Caesar salad wrap Low-fat yogurt with fruit Turkey meatloaf, black bean & corn salad	1,501	468 (31%)

2,000 CALORIES PER DAY			
DAY	DIET	TOTAL CALORIES	PROTEIN CALORIES
MON.	Bagel with cream cheese & lox; orange juice Energy bar Chicken, bean & veggie burrito, grapes Low-fat yogurt with fruit Salmon, brown rice & snow peas (1.5 servings)	1,985	582 (29%)
TUE.	Breakfast wrap; low-fat yogurt with fruit Tuna melt (2 servings); baked snow pea crisps; nectarine Turkey jerky Tofu & vegetable stir-fry (1.5 servings); grapes (1 cup) Soy protein shake	2,017	626 (31%)
WED.	Cereal with skim milk; orange juice Celery sticks with peanut butter Steak wrap; spinach salad; apple Turkey jerky Turkey breast, quinoa & Brussels sprouts (1.5 servings); glass white wine Peach	1,997	582 (29%)
THU.	Vegetable omelet; toasted protein bread with spreadable fruit; orange juice Whey protein shake Turkey sandwich; SunChips; apple Energy bar Pork tenderloins, sweet potato & Swiss chard (1.5 servings) Strawberries	2,003	586 (29%)

Continued on next page

2,000 Calories per Day, *continued*

DAY	DIET	TOTAL CALORIES	PROTEIN CALORIES
FRI.	Protein smoothie; toasted protein bread with spreadable fruit Celery sticks with peanut butter Chicken Caesar salad (1.5 servings); baked snow pea crisps; apple Tuna steak, amaranth & kale Pear	2,006	630 (31%)
SAT.	Egg & veggie scramble; banana; orange juice Soy protein shake; strawberries Lentil & sausage soup (1.5 servings); toasted protein bread with blueberry spreadable fruit Energy bar Chicken & broccoli stir-fry (1.5 servings); glass white wine Peach	1,996	605 (30%)
SUN.	Orange juice Whey protein shake Chicken Caesar salad wrap; pear Low-fat yogurt with fruit Turkey meatloaf, black bean & corn salad (1.5 servings)	2,011	648 (32%)

	2,500 CALORIES PER DAY		
DAY	DIET	TOTAL CALORIES	PROTEIN CALORIES
MON.	Bagel with cream cheese & lox (1.5 servings); orange juice Energy bar; turkey jerky Chicken, bean & veggie burrito, grapes Fruit smoothie with protein Salmon, brown rice & snow peas (1.5 servings) Cherries	2,504	712 (28%)
TUE.	Breakfast wrap; low-fat yogurt with fruit; orange juice Turkey jerky (2 servings) Tuna melt (2 servings); SunChips Fruit smoothie with protein Tofu & vegetable stir-fry (1.5 servings) Soy protein shake; strawberries	2,505	756 (30%)
WED.	Cereal with skim milk (1.5 servings) with ½ sliced banana; orange juice Energy bar Steak wrap (1.5 servings); spinach salad; apple Soy protein shake Turkey breast, quinoa & Brussels sprouts (1.5 servings); glass white wine	2,488	748 (30%)
THU.	Vegetable omelet; toasted protein bread with spreadable fruit; orange juice Soy protein shake with skim milk Turkey sandwich (1.5 servings); baked snow pea crisps; cherries Salmon jerky Pork tenderloins, sweet potato & Swiss chard (2 servings) Energy bar	2,513	764 (30%)

Continued on next page

2,500 Calories per Day, *continued*

DAY	DIET	TOTAL CALORIES	PROTEIN CALORIES
FRI.	Protein smoothie; toasted protein bread with spreadable fruit Celery sticks with peanut butter Chicken Caesar salad (1.5 servings); SunChips; apple Energy bar, strawberries Tuna steak, amaranth & kale (1.5 servings) Pear	2,489	770 (31%)
SAT.	Egg & veggie scramble (2 servings); banana; orange juice Soy protein shake; apple Lentil & sausage soup (1.5 servings); toasted protein bread with blueberry spreadable fruit Celery sticks with peanut butter Chicken & broccoli stir-fry (1.5 servings); glass white wine Low-fat yogurt with fruit	2,492	777 (31%)
SUN.	Orange juice Whey protein shake Chicken Caesar salad wrap (2 servings); pear Low-fat yogurt with fruit Turkey meatloaf, black bean & corn salad (1.5 servings) Pear	2,501	796 (32%)

3,000 CALORIES PER DAY

DAY	DIET	TOTAL CALORIES	PROTEIN CALORIES
MON.	Bagel with cream cheese & lox (1.5 servings); orange juice Energy bar; turkey jerky Chicken, bean & veggie burrito (2 servings); grapes Fruit smoothie with protein Salmon, brown rice & snow peas (1.5 servings) Cherries	2,989	872 (29%)
TUE.	Breakfast wrap (1.5 servings); low-fat yogurt with fruit; orange juice Turkey jerky (2 servings) Tuna melt (2.5 servings); baked snow pea crisps Fruit smoothie with protein Tofu & vegetable stir-fry (2 servings); apple Soy protein shake	3,011	890 (29%)
WED.	Cereal with skim milk (2 servings) with ½ sliced banana; orange juice Energy bar Steak wrap (1.5 servings); spinach salad; apple Soy protein shake; dried fruit medley Turkey breast, quinoa & Brussels sprouts (2 servings); glass white wine	2,998	950 (32%)
THU.	Vegetable omelet (1.5 servings); toasted protein bread with spreadable fruit; orange juice Soy protein shake Turkey sandwich (2 servings); SunChips; cherries Salmon jerky Pork tenderloins, sweet potato & Swiss chard (2 servings); glass white wine Energy bar	3,008	910 (30%)

Continued on next page

3,000 Calories per Day, *continued*

DAY	DIET	TOTAL CALORIES	PROTEIN CALORIES
FRI.	Protein smoothie; toasted protein bread with spreadable fruit Celery sticks with peanut butter (2 servings) Chicken Caesar salad; baked snow pea crisps (2 servings); apple Energy bar, strawberries Tuna steak, amaranth & kale (1.5 servings); glass red wine Low-fat yogurt with fruit	3,004	904 (30%)
SAT.	Egg & veggie scramble (2 servings); banana; orange juice (1.5 servings) Soy protein shake; energy bar Lentil & sausage soup (2 servings); toasted protein bread with blueberry spreadable fruit Celery sticks with peanut butter Chicken & broccoli stir-fry (2 servings); glass white wine; apple Low-fat yogurt with fruit	2,991	894 (30%)
SUN.	Orange juice Whey protein shake Chicken Caesar salad wrap (2 servings); pear Low-fat yogurt with fruit Turkey meatloaf, black bean & corn salad (1.5 servings); glass white wine Apple	3,004	916 (30%)

VEGETARIAN MEAL PLAN

This is a one-day example of a meal plan appropriate for vegetarians aiming to consume roughly 2,375 calories per day in a Racing Weight quick start. While this number may seem arbitrary in comparison to the other meal plans, keep in mind that the individual daily calorie target you come up with using the method I've shown you is very unlikely to be a nice round number (e.g., 2,000 calories). So this example represents a more likely scenario.

VEGETARIAN: 2,375 CALORIES PER DAY		
DIET	TOTAL CALORIES	PROTEIN CALORIES
Cereal with almond milk (2 servings); orange juice	2,375	654 (27%)
Soy protein shake; apple		
Lentil soup; peanut butter & jelly sandwich on protein bread		
Soy protein shake		
Tofu & vegetable stir-fry with brown rice (2 servings)		
Cherries		

QUICK START TRAINING

There are two objectives to the training you do within a Racing Weight quick start. The first is to perform workouts that cooperate with your diet to make you leaner. The second is to establish a solid sport-specific fitness foundation to build upon after you complete the quick start and begin your race-focused training cycle. To maximize your success in pursuit of these two objectives you need to train somewhat differently than you would if you were just pursuing one or the other. The special quick start training approach I will outline in this chapter represents the best way to simultaneously maximize fat loss and build foundational fitness for your sport.

Your quick start training will include three types of workouts: high-intensity interval sessions, prolonged fat-burning workouts, and strength workouts. Short (10–30-second) intervals of maximum or near-maximum intensity contribute to fat loss by creating a huge post-workout fat-burning effect. At the same time, high-intensity intervals help prepare the body for race-focused training by increasing raw speed and power that will in turn enable you to perform all your subsequent training at a higher level. For endurance athletes, speed and power play a much smaller role later in training when the focus shifts to race-specific training, which should include longer intervals. Intervals lasting more than a minute each will be more productive later in your training because, to be done most effectively, these workouts require a higher level of calorie and carbohydrate intake than you will have during a quick start. They are also more effective when you've laid down a solid foundation of fitness beforehand, as you will do in your quick start.

Prolonged fat-burning workouts contribute to fat loss by maximizing fat burning within the sessions themselves and by increasing your muscles' capacity to burn fat. No other type of workout burns more fat than a long one performed at a steady, moderate intensity, especially when the workout is conducted in a carbohydrate-deprived state. Prolonged fat-burning workouts also prepare your body for future race-focused training by developing your raw endurance in a gentle way. Your ultimate goal in racing is to sustain a high rate of speed for a prolonged period of time. To do that you must first perform some lengthy workouts at challenging tempos. But before you do that you must prepare your body to handle such challenging race-specific workouts by performing longer workouts at more relaxed speeds. That's where prolonged fat-burning workouts come in; their function is to give you more than enough endurance to merely "go the distance" in races so you can then work on sustaining greater speeds over distance.

Strength training contributes to fat loss by increasing muscle mass and with it your body's resting metabolic rate, so your body burns more fat around the clock. It also prepares your body for the training cycle by making you stronger. Raw muscle strength is undervalued by most endurance athletes. The stronger you can get without sacrificing endurance, speed, and technique, the better you will perform as a cyclist, runner, or triathlete. Obviously, if you were to quit cycling, running, and/or swimming in favor of lifting weights for two hours every day, you would get a lot stronger but your sport performance would suffer due to loss of endurance, speed, and technique. Maximizing strength without sacrificing these attributes requires a balancing act in training. One way to maintain the right balance is to mix a modest amount of strength training with a greater amount of sport-specific endurance training throughout the training cycle. But you can achieve further benefit by making strength training a higher priority before the training cycle begins. Focusing on strength training in a quick start allows you to get stronger than you ever could if you never prioritized strength training, yet it does not interfere with your race fitness development because this strength-focus period falls before the start of the formal training cycle.

Let's take a closer look at how you will implement high-intensity intervals, prolonged fat-burning workouts, and strength workouts in your quick start.

HIGH-INTENSITY INTERVALS

It's not surprising that high-intensity intervals are a more time-efficient way to stimulate fat loss than steady, moderate-intensity workouts. Obviously, the more intensely you exercise, the more calories you burn per minute. Therefore, a high-intensity interval workout of a given duration always stimulates more fat loss than a steady, moderate-intensity workout of equal duration. But it might surprise you to learn that, in addition to stimulating more fat loss when time is held constant, high-intensity intervals also stimulate more fat loss when the total energy cost of the two types of workouts is held constant. For example, a previously sedentary person who starts an exercise program in which she burns 400 calories per day in high-intensity interval workouts will probably lose more body fat than she would if she started an exercise program in which she burned exactly the same number of calories in steady, moderate-intensity workouts (which, of course, would take longer to complete than the interval workouts). The reason is that the new exerciser would burn a lot more fat between high-intensity interval workouts than between steady, moderate-intensity workouts.

Experts on the use of high-intensity intervals for fat loss, including Martin Gibala at McMaster University, favor very short, maximum- or near-maximum-intensity intervals (10 to 30 seconds) to stimulate fat loss in obese and low-fitness individuals. Even though these sessions are very hard, they are generally more tolerable to beginners than the sorts of intervals more often practiced by endurance athletes, which are still very intense but last much longer (1 to 5 minutes). The average sedentary person can get through a bunch of 10- or 30-second sprints separated by plenty of recovery time without experiencing undue misery, but a handful of 3-minute supra-threshold intervals would be hell on earth.

In addition to being the best form of interval training for obese and low-fitness individuals, these very short, very high-intensity intervals are also the best form of interval training for endurance athletes within a quick start. That's because sprints are not only more manageable than longer intervals for the beginner but also more manageable for the experienced endurance athlete who is relatively far from peak fitness at the moment, and endurance athletes typically are farthest from peak fitness in the several weeks before they begin a new training cycle. And again, by developing reserves of raw speed and power, this type of training does a good job of preparing athletes for the base training period that comes at the start of a new training cycle.

The most appropriate way to approach quick start interval training varies by sport. Here are some guidelines for cyclists, runners, and triathletes.

CYCLISTS

There are three types of near-maximum- to maximum-intensity intervals you can do on the bike: speed intervals, power intervals, and short hill intervals. Speed intervals emphasize leg turnover. They entail sprinting at a very high cadence in a moderate gear. Power intervals emphasize pushing against resistance. The intensity is the same as in speed intervals—both are all-out efforts—but power intervals are performed in your bike's highest gear (outdoors) or against very high resistance (indoors). Short hill intervals are short maximum-intensity hill climbs performed out of the saddle on a moderately steep (5–8 percent) grade.

► HIGH-INTENSITY INTERVALS DEVELOP RESERVES OF RAW POWER AND SPEED TO PREPARE ATHLETES FOR THE BASE TRAINING PERIOD THAT FOLLOWS THE QUICK START.

The metabolic benefits of the three interval types are the same. In other words, each will stimulate about the same amount of fat loss as the others. There are slight differences, though, in the fitness and performance benefits of the three workouts. As you might expect, speed intervals do the best job of enhancing maximum cadence and efficiency at very high cadences, power intervals do the best job of increasing maximal power output, and short hill sprints do the best job of enhancing hill-climbing ability.

Here are example formats of each workout type:

Speed Intervals

Warm up with 10–15 minutes of easy spinning. Ride 12 x 30 seconds at maximal effort (that is, the greatest effort you can sustain through all 12 intervals) at 120+ rpm in a gear that is slightly below the preferred gear. Spin for 1 minute after each sprint. Cool down with 10–15 minutes of easy spinning.

Power Intervals

Warm up with 10–15 minutes of easy spinning. Ride 20 x 10 seconds at maximal effort (that is, the greatest effort you can sustain through all 20 intervals) in your highest gear or at whatever resistance level yields the highest power output on your indoor bike. (Power intervals are indeed best done on an indoor bike.) Spin for 1 minute after each interval. Cool down with 10–15 minutes of easy spinning.

Short Hill Intervals

Warm up with 10–15 minutes of easy spinning. Ride 16 x 20 seconds at maximal effort (that is, the greatest effort you can sustain through all 16 intervals) out of the saddle on a moderately steep (5–7 percent) hill.

Coast back down the hill and spin for 1 minute after each interval. Cool down with 10–15 minutes of easy spinning.

RUNNERS

Sprinting on level ground is very stressful on the muscles and tendons. For this reason, I seldom prescribe it. You can get the strength, speed, power, and fat-loss benefits you seek from maximum-intensity running with less chance of injury if you sprint uphill instead. Hill sprints (10-second efforts) and hill intervals (20- to 30-second efforts) together represent one of two types of interval training I recommend for runners in a quick start.

The other type is indoor cycling power intervals as described above. Cycling intervals for runners? That's right. The reason I have runners perform power intervals on a bike instead of on foot is that a running workout that yields the equivalent neuromuscular and metabolic stimuli would leave you unable to get out of bed the next day. Legs are legs. The power that the cycling workout creates in your legs will transfer over to your running. And fat burning is fat burning. As a runner you will burn just as much fat with cycling power intervals as a cyclist. Of course, no alternative form of exercise offers as much running-specific fitness benefit as running itself, but you will do plenty of running in your quick start. This cross-training workout will complement that running to provide more of the special benefits you seek in a quick start than any type of additional run would do.

Here are some examples of hill sprint and hill interval workout formats.

Hill Sprints

Run 45 minutes easy. Sprint 8 x 10 seconds up a moderately steep to steep hill (5–10 percent grade). Walk back down the hill to recover after each sprint. Hill sprints should always follow an easy run because an easy run serves as a good warm-up for sprints. Furthermore, it's unlikely that you will ever do enough hill sprints to make a complete workout of them.

Hill Intervals

Warm up with 10 minutes of easy running. Run 12 x 30 seconds uphill at the greatest speed you can sustain through the last interval. Jog slowly back down the hill for recovery. Cool down with 10 minutes of easy running.

TRIATHLETES

As a triathlete you will do the same high-intensity cycling interval sessions cyclists do and the same high-intensity running sessions runners do, but you will also do high-intensity swim intervals. High-intensity intervals are not as special in swimming as they are in cycling and running, because swimming is much gentler on the musculoskeletal system; therefore speed and power work is less stressful and easier to recover from when done in the water. Consequently, triathletes traditionally do much more high-intensity interval work in the pool than they do on the bike or on foot. Still, I recommend that triathletes approach their swim training differently in a quick start than at other times, specifically by focusing more on the shortest sprints and on strength work with fins and paddles (separately).

Following are some examples of short sprint sets, kick sets with fins, and pull sets with paddles. All three can be incorporated into a single workout, but they can also be done in separate workouts or together in any combination of two of the three.

Sprint Set

12 x 25 yards/meters at maximum speed. Recover 10 seconds.

Kick Set

12 x 25 yards/meters kicking on sides with fins. Recover 10 seconds.

Pull Set

10 x 50 yards/meters pulling with small paddles. Recover 15 seconds.

PROLONGED FAT-BURNING WORKOUTS

If high-intensity interval sessions are the most efficient workouts for fat loss, why would you ever do any other types of workouts? Three reasons. First, high-intensity interval rides and runs are very stressful and cannot be done every day. But you need to train every day, so it's necessary to do some other types of workouts between interval sessions.

Second, while high-intensity interval workouts are the most efficient means to stimulate fat loss, they are not the only means, nor are they necessarily the most potent. Extended moderate-intensity workouts stimulate fat loss in ways that are largely complementary to the ways in which high-intensity intervals stimulate fat loss, so it's best to do both. Specifically, high-intensity intervals deplete your muscle carbohydrate stores, causing your body to burn a significant amount of fat *after* the workout, while your carbohydrate stores are being replenished, whereas longer moderate-intensity workouts burn lots of fat within the workouts themselves and cultivate your muscles' general fat-burning capacity. Also, even though high-intensity intervals stimulate more fat loss than steady, moderate-intensity workouts, when either the duration or the total energy cost of the two workout types is held constant, moderate-intensity training ultimately has greater potential to stimulate fat loss. You can go much longer at a moderate intensity and thus greatly exceed the maximum energy cost you can achieve with an exhaustive interval workout.

A third reason not to rely on high-intensity intervals exclusively in a quick start is that fat burning is not the only goal of the training you do within a quick start. Remember, your other objective is to lay a foundation of sport-specific fitness to build on later. As an endurance athlete, you need the endurance you get from prolonged fat-burning

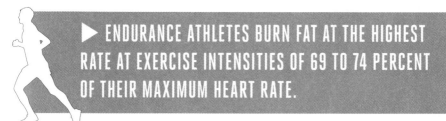

▶ ENDURANCE ATHLETES BURN FAT AT THE HIGHEST RATE AT EXERCISE INTENSITIES OF 69 TO 74 PERCENT OF THEIR MAXIMUM HEART RATE.

intensity workouts as much as you need the speed and power you get from high-intensity intervals.

Research has shown that trained endurance athletes burn fat at the highest rate at exercise intensities of 69 to 74 percent of their maximum heart rate.[1] So this is the intensity you'll want to target in prolonged fat-burning workouts. If you don't use a heart rate monitor, don't sweat it. Fat burning hovers within 10 percent of the maximal rate through a broad spectrum of intensity levels, from about 65 to 82 percent of maximum heart rate, and it's pretty easy to find that range by feel. For the fit individual, it's an intensity that feels very comfortable but not dawdling. The mistake you most want to avoid in these workouts is going too fast, because the rate of fat burning drops precipitously at intensities above 82 percent of maximum heart rate as carbohydrate burning takes over. Keep the following mantra in the back of your mind when doing prolonged fat-burning workouts: Cruise, don't push.

Even within the so-called fat-burning intensity range, fat burning is suppressed when carbohydrates are consumed during the workout. Your muscles are smart enough to use the fast extra energy provided by the carbs in a sports drink or energy gel in preference to body fat when given the opportunity. Therefore you are not to consume any carbs during the prolonged fat-burning workouts in your quick start. In fact, ideally you will not consume any carbs within several hours before these workouts either, because fat burning is truly maximized when your muscles are already in a carbohydrate-depleted state at the start of the workout. For most athletes, the most practical way to train in a fasted state is to do the workout early in the morning without a preceding breakfast.

If you've never done this type of workout before, be prepared. You will probably feel lethargic and, well, lousy the first few times as your muscles struggle to keep the "furnace" stoked for an hour or more with nothing but "low-octane" intramuscular triglycerides and free fatty acids. But after surviving a few such sessions you will begin to

---

1   J. Achten, M. Gleeson, and A. E. Jeukendrup, "Determination of the Exercise Intensity That Elicits Maximal Fat Oxidation," *Medicine & Science in Sports & Exercise* 34, no. 1 (January 2002): 92–7.

feel more comfortable in them, and that's a sign that your muscles are indeed becoming better fat burners.

"Prolonged" is always a relative term in endurance training. Advanced athletes can handle longer workouts than beginners, long-distance racers require longer endurance-building sessions than short-distance racers, and cycling is more conducive to prolonged training than running. Prolonged fat-burning workouts need to last at least 60 minutes, preferably at least 90, to fulfill their purpose, so I encourage even relative beginners and short-distance racers to push beyond the hour mark. Because the intensity is moderate, it's not so hard. At the same time, it is not necessary or even advisable to cover epic distances in these workouts because the carbohydrate deprivation will greatly reduce your normal range.

Following are prolonged fat-burning workout guidelines for cyclists, runners, and triathletes. They're pretty simple.

Fat-Burning Workouts for Cyclists

First thing in the morning, without eating breakfast, hop on your bike and ride 90 minutes to 3 hours at 65 to 75 percent of your maximum heart rate, drinking only water or a zero-calorie electrolyte solution as you go.

Fat-Burning Workouts for Runners

First thing in the morning, without eating breakfast, run 1 to 2.5 hours at 65 to 75 percent of your maximum heart rate, drinking only water or a zero-calorie electrolyte solution as you go.

Fat-Burning Workouts for Triathletes

Perform one prolonged fat-burning ride and one prolonged fat-burning run every other week in alternate weeks. Also do a longer, steady, moderate-intensity swim each week. The swim workout does not need to be performed in a fasted state, however, nor does it need to last a full hour.

STRENGTH WORKOUTS

Most endurance athletes do not love lifting weights. Knowing this, I design the simplest and most time-efficient strength workouts possible for endurance athletes for all circumstances, including quick starts. All the strength workouts included in the training plans in the next three chapters share the same basic format: 10 total exercises, including three each for the lower body, core, and upper body, arranged in repeating lower body/core/upper body sequences, with one extra lower-body exercise tacked onto the end.

The least challenging version of this workout requires that each exercise be performed just once. The more challenging versions require that each exercise be performed twice or even three times in a circuit format, meaning you do each exercise once, then go back and do it a second time, and so on. All the training plans include two to three strength workouts per week.

The specific exercises included in the workouts vary from sport to sport and from week to week. The cycling plans include those exercises I judge best for cyclists, the running plans are built from the most beneficial exercises for runners, and the triathlon plans combine these with the best exercises for swimmers. The strength workouts in all the plans are dominated by basic bodyweight exercises in the first week, then gradually introduce more advanced exercises involving external resistance in subsequent weeks.

Following are descriptions and illustrations of all the exercises used in the quick start strength workouts. Note that recommendations for the number of repetitions will be given within the training plans themselves in the next three chapters. Some of the exercises involve a form of external resistance (dumbbells, cable pulley weight stacks, etc.) while others do not, and still others may be done either way. For those exercises where external resistance is optional or required, choose a level of resistance appropriate for the designated number of repetitions. Specifically, chose a resistance level that leaves you significantly fatigued but not exhausted at the end of a set, able to complete one or two more repetitions if you had to but no more.

LOWER BODY

These 15 exercises target the hips, groin, gluteals, quadriceps, hamstrings, calves, and feet. Some also have secondary benefits for the core and upper body.

BALANCING BEND AND REACH
Feet, calves, hamstrings, glutes, hips, quads

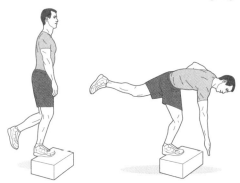

Stand on your right foot on the edge of a box or other sturdy support with your forefoot supported and your heel dangling off the edge. Your left leg is slightly bent to elevate your left foot. Bend at the waist, hip, and knee and reach toward the floor in front of you with your right hand. Extend your left leg behind your body for balance as you bend and reach. Stretch your fingertips as close to the floor as you can get them without losing balance. Return to the start position. Complete a full set and then repeat the exercise standing on your left leg.

BALANCE BALL LEG CURL
Hamstrings

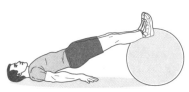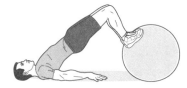

Lie on your back and place your heels together on top of a stability ball. Raise your pelvis so that your body forms a straight plank from head to toes. Contract your gluteal muscles and hamstrings and roll the ball toward your body. Pause briefly and return to the start position. Focus on keeping your pelvis from sagging toward the floor throughout this movement. To make this exercise more challenging, perform single-leg curls with one heel on the ball and the other foot elevated a few inches above it.

ECCENTRIC HEEL DIP

Calves

Balance on one foot on a sturdy platform such as an aerobics step, with the ball of the foot resting on the edge of the platform so that the heel is unsupported and hanging off the back of the platform. Rest your fingertips against a wall or some other support for balance. Lower your heel toward the floor until you feel a stretch 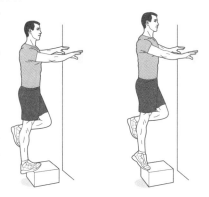 in your calf muscles. (Your heel will now be below the level of the ball of your foot.) Then raise your heel back to a neutral position. At first, when you lift your body back to the starting position, do so with both legs so that you are not overloading the calf muscles. Once you're stronger, you may attempt the lifting phase with one calf. Always use one for the lowering phase. Complete a full set and then work the other calf.

ELEVATED REVERSE LUNGE

Hips, groin, gluteals, quadriceps, hamstrings

Stand on a 4- to 6-inch step with your arms resting at your sides and a dumbbell in each hand. Take a big step backward with one leg and bend both knees until the back foot hits the ground and the back knee almost grazes the floor. Now forcefully contract the quads and gluteals of your forward leg to draw your rear leg forward and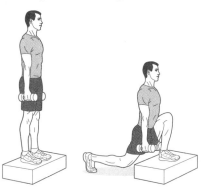

EXERCISES

your body back to a standing position. Be sure to maintain an upright torso posture throughout the movement. Complete a full set with one leg, rest, then work the opposite leg.

GIANT WALKING LUNGE
Hips, gluteals, quadriceps, hamstrings

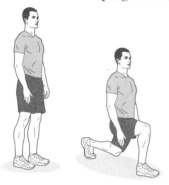

Walk slowly forward by taking the longest steps possible. With each new step, imagine you're trying to break your "personal record" for the largest step you've ever taken. Keep your arms relaxed at your sides. If this is not challenging, perform the exercise with a dumbbell in each hand.

GLUTEAL-HAMSTRING RAISE
Gluteals, hamstrings

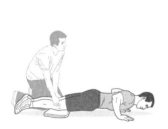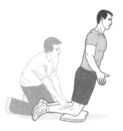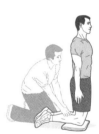

Lie on your stomach and have a partner press your lower legs down into the floor so your body can only move from the knees up. With your arms in standard push-up position, give a slight push off the floor while you contract your hamstrings and gluteals and lift your body (from knees to head) upward until you are in a fully upright kneeling position. Try to keep your torso aligned with your thighs (don't bend at the waist) throughout the movement. Lower yourself back to the floor.

HIP HIKE

Hips

Stand on your left foot on a sturdy platform that's at least eight inches high. Position yourself so that the instep of your foot is close to the edge of the platform and your right foot is hovering above the floor. Begin with your hips aligned so your right foot is level with your left. Now relax the muscles of your left hip and allow

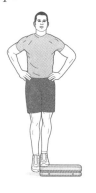
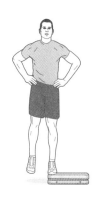

your right foot to sink a few inches toward the floor. Be sure to do this without bending your left knee. Next, contract the muscles of your left hip and lift your right hip as high as possible, bringing your right foot a few inches higher than the left. Complete a full set and then reverse your position and repeat the exercise.

KETTLEBELL SQUAT SWING

Gluteals, quadriceps, hamstrings, abs,
lower back, upper back, shoulders

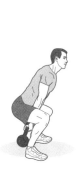
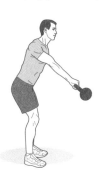
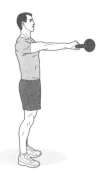

Stand with your feet slightly wider than shoulder-width apart, knees bent roughly 15 degrees, toes turned out slightly, and a kettlebell placed on the floor between your feet. Bend over and grab the kettlebell with both hands, then return your torso to a fully upright position, keeping your arms fully extended toward the floor in front of your body so the kettlebell is between your upper thighs. To start the exercise, bend your torso forward from the hips (not the waist) and swing the kettlebell backward between your legs as though you're preparing to take a "diaper shot" with a basketball. Next, with a fluid, powerful motion, extend your hips and shoulders, swinging the kettlebell upward and forward until it reaches the level of your shoulders in a standing position. Now reverse this movement, bending forward, lowering your arms and allowing the kettlebell to swing back through your legs. If you don't have access to a kettlebell, use a dumbbell, holding it by one end with both hands.

ROMANIAN DEADLIFT

Hamstrings, lower back

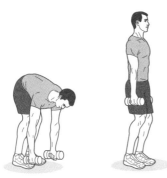

Stand with your feet close together, knees bent very slightly, with a dumbbell next to each foot. Bend forward at the waist and grab the dumbbells. With arms at your sides and knees locked in a slightly bent position, return to a standing position. Pause briefly and then bend forward to do another repetition.

SINGLE-LEG SQUAT

Hips, gluteals, quadriceps, hamstrings

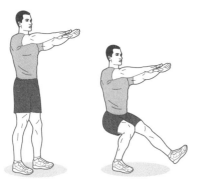

Stand on your right foot and bend the left leg slightly to elevate the left foot a few inches above the floor. Lower your posterior slowly toward the floor, keeping most of your weight on the heel of your support foot. Reach the left leg either behind your body (easier) or in front of your body (harder) to keep it out of the way and to help maintain balance. Squat as low as you can go without your pelvis swinging outward. Return to the start position. Complete a full set and then repeat the exercise on your left foot.

SPLIT SQUAT JUMP

Quadriceps, hamstrings, gluteals, calves, hips

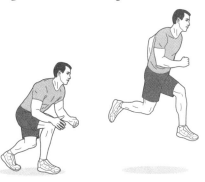

Start in a split stance with your right foot flat on the ground and your left leg slightly bent with only the forefoot of your left foot touching the ground a half step behind the right. Lower yourself into a deep squat and then leap upward as high as possible. In midair, reverse the position of your legs. When you land, sink down immediately into another squat and then leap again. Use your arms for balance and to generate extra upward thrust with each leap.

SPLIT-STANCE DUMBBELL DEADLIFT

Gluteals, hips, hamstrings, quadriceps, lower back, upper back

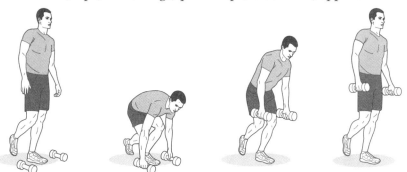

Stand with your left foot directly beneath your left hip and your right foot half a step behind the right hip with only the toe touching the floor. Put all your weight on your left foot; use the right only for balance. Begin with a dumbbell positioned on the floor directly underneath your hands as your arms hang at your sides. Bend down and grab the dumbbells. Press your left foot into the floor and stand fully upright. Concentrate on extending your left knee and hip first and then lifting your torso. Keep your weight fully on your left foot throughout this movement. Pause briefly in a standing position and then lower the dumbbells back to the floor. Complete a full set, then reverse your position and do another set.

STEP-UP
Quadriceps, hamstrings, hips, groin, gluteals

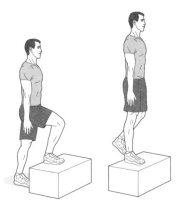

Stand facing a sturdy 12- to 18-inch platform such as an aerobic step with your right foot on it and your left foot on the floor. Now use your right leg to pull your body upward until you're standing on the bench on your right foot. Concentrate on not pushing off the floor with your left foot. (One way to ensure you do this is to lift the toes of your left foot before you engage your right leg to lift your body.) Make your right leg do all the work of lifting your body. Step back down with your left leg. Repeat until you've completed a full set, then switch legs.

SUPINE GLUTEAL ACTIVATION
Gluteals, abs

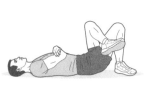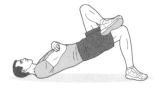

Lie on your back with your right leg bent 90 degrees and your right foot flat on the floor close to your posterior. Begin with your left knee sharply bent and crossed over the right leg so that the lateral side of your left ankle is resting against your lower right thigh. Your hands are folded on your chest. Now contract your right gluteals and lift your hip until your right thigh and torso form a straight line. Concentrate on using your gluteals more than your hamstrings to achieve this lifting. Pause one second with your hip elevated and return to the start position. Complete a full set, then reverse your position and repeat the exercise.

X-BAND WALK
Hips, groin

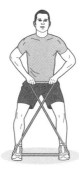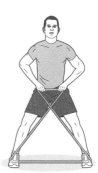

Loop a half-inch or one-inch exercise band under both feet and stand on top of it. Your feet should be roughly 12 inches apart at the start. Cross the ends of the band to form an X and grasp one end in each hand. Pull your chest up and shoulders back, keeping tension on the band throughout the ensuing movement. Start walking sideways with small lateral steps. The leg that's on the side of the direction you're moving will have to overcome the band's tension to take each step. Make sure you keep the hips and shoulders level, and don't deviate forward or backward as you step to the side. When this exercise is performed correctly, you'll feel the movement in your gluteals. Complete 10 steps in one direction, then 10 more moving in the opposite direction.

CORE

These seven exercises target various parts of the abdominal region and the lower back. Some have secondary benefits for other areas.

L-OVER
Abs, obliques

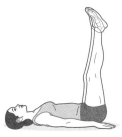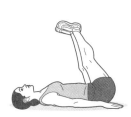

Lie on your back with your arms resting at your sides and your palms flat on the floor. Extend your legs directly toward the ceiling, touch your feet together, and point your toes. Keeping your big toes together, tip your legs 12 to 18 inches to the left by twisting at the hips, so that your right buttock comes off the floor. Fight the pull of gravity by maintaining stability with your abdominals and obliques. Pause for a moment, then return slowly to the start position, again using your core muscles to control the movement. Repeat on the right side, and continue alternating from left to right until you've completed a full set.

ALTERNATING SINGLE-LEG REVERSE CRUNCH
Abs, hip flexors

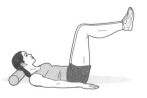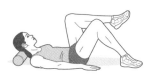

Lie on your back with your head supported by a large pillow or foam roller. Begin with your legs bent 90 degrees and your thighs perpendicular to the floor, feet together. Engage your deep abs by drawing your navel toward your spine and trying to flatten your lower back against the floor. While holding this contraction, slowly lower your right foot to the floor. Return immediately to the start position, and then lower the left foot. If you find this movement easy, you are failing to hold the contraction of your deep abs. Keep your back pressed so flat to the floor that a credit card couldn't be squeezed between them! Lower each foot to the floor 8 to 10 times.

PLANK
Abs, lower back

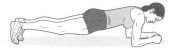 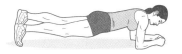

Lie on the floor on your stomach, with your upper body supported on your forearms and your toes pressing into the ground. Maintain a 90-degree bend in your elbows and make sure they are placed directly underneath the shoulders. Tighten your entire core area and lift your hips up and in line with your legs and torso. Hold this position for up to 30 seconds without allowing your hips to sag. If you can hold the prone plank position longer than 30 seconds, make this exercise more challenging by doing it with your left foot elevated a few inches above the floor for 15 seconds, then your right foot elevated for 15 seconds.

REVERSE PLANK
Abs

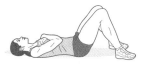 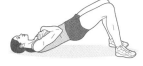

Lie on your back on the floor with your arms folded on your chest, your knees bent 90 degrees, and your feet flat on the floor. Contract your gluteals and lift your hips until your body forms a straight line from neck to knees. Hold this position.

EXERCISES

SIDE PLANK
Abs, obliques, hips

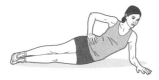 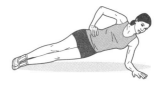

Lie on your left side with your ankles together and your torso propped up by your upper arm. Lift your hips upward until your body forms a diagonal plank from ankles to neck. Hold this position for 20 to 30 seconds, making sure you don't allow your hips to sag toward the floor. (Watch yourself in a mirror to make sure you're not sagging.) Switch to the left side and repeat the exercise.

STICK CRUNCH
Abs

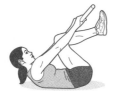 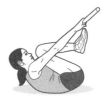

Lie on your back, bend your knees, and draw them as close to your chest as possible. Grasp any type of stick or rod (such as a broom handle) with both hands, positioned shoulder-width apart. Begin with your arms extended straight toward your toes, your abs tightened, and your head and upper back curled slightly off the floor. Now squeeze your abdominal muscles and reach forward with the stick until it passes beyond your toes. (This is a very small movement—just a few inches.) Pause for one second and return to the start position. Don't allow your abs to completely relax.

EXERCISES

SUITCASE DEADLIFT
Obliques, hips, lower back, upper back,
gluteals, hamstrings, quadriceps

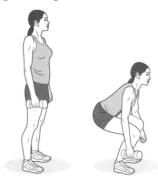

Stand with your arms hanging at your sides and a dumbbell in one hand. Push your hips back, bend the knees, and reach the dumbbell down as close to the floor as you can while maintaining a neutral spine (some people have a tendency to round their back at the bottom of this movement). Now stand up again. Don't allow your torso to tilt to either side while performing this movement. Complete a full set, rest for 30 seconds, then repeat the exercise while holding the dumbbell in the opposite hand.

UPPER BODY

These nine exercises target the shoulders, chest, upper back, and arms. Some have secondary benefits for other parts.

BENT-OVER CABLE SHOULDER LATERAL EXTENSION
Shoulders, upper back

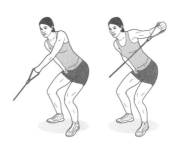

Stand in a wide stance with your knees slightly bent and your right side facing a cable pulley station with a D-handle connected to the low attachment point. Grasp the handle in your left hand using an underhand grip. Bend forward 45 degrees from the hips. Begin with your left arm extended toward the floor and the handle positioned directly underneath your breastbone. Tighten your core. Now pull the handle outward and upward until your left arm is fully extended away from your body and parallel to the floor. Pause briefly and return to the start position. Complete a full set, then reverse your position and work the right shoulder.

CABLE EXTERNAL SHOULDER ROTATION
Shoulders

There are two versions of this exercise: neutral rotation and overhead rotation.

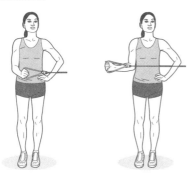

Neutral Rotation: Stand with your left side facing a cable pulley station. Grasp the handle in your right hand and begin with your right arm bent 90 degrees so that your forearm is pointing toward the cable pulley station across your belly. Now rotate your shoulder externally and pull the handle across your body. Return to the start position. Complete a full set and repeat the exercise with your left arm.

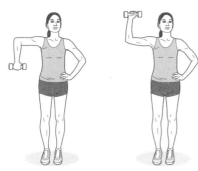

Overhead Rotation: Stand with your right upper arm extended away from your body at shoulder level, your elbow bent 90 degrees, and your shoulder rotated internally so your forearm is pointing toward the floor. Hold a small dumbbell in your right hand. Now rotate your shoulder externally 180 degrees, stopping when your right forearm is pointing toward the ceiling. Return to the start position. Complete a full set and repeat the exercise with your left arm.

CABLE FACE PULL
Shoulders, upper back

Set up a pulley with the rope attachment just above forehead level. Stand facing the pulley in a split stance and hold the rope with a neutral grip (palms facing in). Your arms are extended straight out in front of you with the hands slightly above shoulder height. Pull the center of the rope attachment toward your forehead 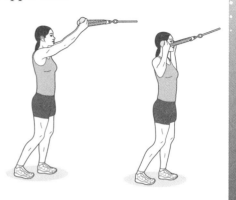 by retracting the shoulder blades and forcing the elbows out (not down). As the rope approaches your face, your shoulder blades should be pulled back and down, with the chest high and your hands coming even with your ears. You should feel the resistance in your mid back and in the back of your shoulders.

CHIN-UP
Upper back, arms, shoulders

Begin by hanging from a chin-up bar with an underhand grip on the bar and your hands positioned slightly farther than shoulder-width apart. Pull your body upward toward the bar until your chin is at bar level. Pause briefly and slowly lower yourself back to the start position.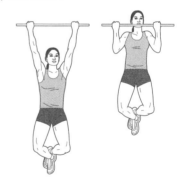

If you cannot complete at least eight chin-ups, do a modified chin-up. Set a Smith machine barbell at a height of three to four feet above the floor. Sit under the bar and grab it underhand with your hands positioned at shoulder width. Raise your hips up and form a straight line with your whole body. You are now "hanging" from the bar with only your heels touching the floor. Pull your chest to the bar and then return slowly to a hanging position.

HALF-KNEEL CABLE PULL

Chest, upper back, shoulders, lower back, abs, obliques

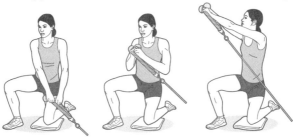

Assume a half-kneel position with your left knee and your right foot on the floor. You may want to place a pad under your knee for comfort. Position yourself three feet away from a cable pulley station with your torso facing it at a 45-degree angle. Attach a V-rope to the cable at ankle height. Grab a segment of the rope in each hand. Begin with your arms fully extended toward the attachment point. Pull your hands to your chest, pause briefly, and then extend your arms fully upward and away from your body. The cable should move in the same line in both parts of this movement. In other words, when you extend your arms in the second part of the movement, the cable should continue to move in exactly the same direction it did when you pulled your hands to your chest. After extending your arms fully, pause briefly once more and then return to the start position in one fluid movement. Your torso should not rotate while performing this exercise. Complete a full set, then reverse your stance and do another set.

INVERTED SHOULDER PRESS

Shoulders, arms, chest

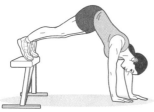 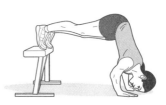

Assume a push-up position but with your feet elevated on an exercise bench or other sturdy platform of similar height. Position your hands close enough to your feet so your body forms an inverted V with a 60

to 90 degree bend at the waist. Bend your elbows and lower the top of your head toward the floor between your hands, stopping just short of making contact. Press back to the start position. The higher you elevate your feet and the more you bend at the waist, the more challenging this exercise will be.

ONE-ARM DUMBBELL SNATCH

Shoulders, upper back, arms, lower back,
gluteals, quadriceps, hamstrings

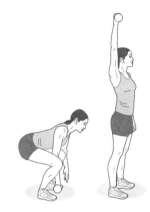

Stand in a wide stance with a single dumbbell placed on the floor between your feet. Bend your knees, tilt forward from the hips, and grasp the dumbbell with your right hand using an overhand grip (knuckles facing forward). Begin with your right arm fully extended. The object of this exercise is to lift the dumbbell in a straight line from the floor to a point directly overhead. To do this, begin by contracting your gluteals, hamstrings, and lower back so that the dumbbell rises to thigh height as you assume an upright standing position. From this point, keep the dumbbell moving in a straight line close to your body by bending your elbow and pulling from the shoulder. As the dumbbell approaches head level, rotate your shoulder and extend your arm until it is pointing toward the ceiling. Pause briefly, then reverse the movement, allowing the dumbbell to come to rest again on the floor briefly before initiating the next lift. Complete a full set, then switch to the left arm.

PUSH PRESS

Shoulders, gluteals, hamstrings, quadriceps

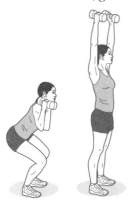

Stand with a dumbbell in each hand and your elbows fully flexed so the weights are at your shoulders. Your palms are facing each other and your feet are shoulder-width apart. Bend your knees and lower yourself into a half-squat. Immediately reverse this movement, powerfully straightening your legs and hips. As soon as you're once again fully upright, press the dumbbells straight overhead. The idea is to use the upward momentum created by straightening your legs to assist your shoulders and arms in pushing the dumbbells toward the ceiling. This allows you to lift more weight than you could with a standard shoulder press. (But keep the weight light until you've mastered the movement.)

To complete the movement, lower the dumbbells back down to your shoulders.

PUSH-UP

Chest, upper back, shoulders, arms, abs, lower back

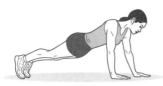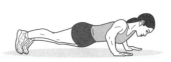

Assume a standard push-up position with your hands just outside shoulder width. Imagine your body being a straight line from ankles to neck; don't allow the hips to sag or your butt to stick up too high. Tuck your chin so that your head is close to being in line with your body. Lower your chest to within an inch of the floor. Look straight at the floor the entire time and keep your core braced tightly. Press back to the starting position.

If you can't do at least 10 standard push-ups, instead do elevated push-ups with your hands positioned on an exercise bench. If you can do more than 20 push-ups, instead do resisted push-ups with a resistance band wrapped over your shoulder blades and the ends pressed to the floor under your hands.

Strength training is something you should do not only during a quick start but also throughout the training cycle. Your time commitment to strength training should be somewhat less during the training cycle, though. See *Racing Weight* for strength workouts appropriate for race-focused training periods.

SEVEN

TRAINING PLANS
FOR CYCLISTS

D o you race bikes or participate in long non-competitive cycling events ? If so, here are your quick start training plans. The "low-volume" plans are a good choice if you are less fit, less experienced, or simply have less time on your hands. The "high-volume" plans are ideal if you have a good degree of fitness and experience and some extra time to work out. Once you decide which plan suits you, it's time to choose how long your quick start will be: four, six, or eight weeks. As I have mentioned previously, I recommend that you do a four-week quick start if you are within 10 lbs. of your racing weight, a six-week quick start if you are 11 to 20 lbs. above your racing weight, and an eight-week quick start if you are more than 20 lbs. above your racing weight.

The six- and eight-week plans are extended versions of the four-week plan, so only two schedules are presented. If you choose to follow the four-week low-volume plan, for example, just complete the

the workouts in the first four weeks of the low-volume schedule and then move on to your race-focused training. The low-volume plans feature six workouts per week: four rides and two strength workouts. The high-volume plans feature six rides and three strength workouts. The low-volume plans start with just over 3 hours of riding and roughly 4 hours of total training in Week 1 and peak at nearly 5 hours of riding and 7 hours of total training in Week 8. The high-volume plans start with close to 8 hours of riding and close to 9 hours of total training in Week 1 and peak at approximately 10 hours of riding and 13 hours of total training in Week 7. (Week 8 has a slightly lighter load than Week 7 because it includes a rest day.)

You should feel free to tweak your chosen plan to suit your schedule and specific needs. Don't mess with it too much, however. Resist temptations to do significantly longer Fat-Burning Rides because you worry they will not be challenging enough (they will be, because of your fasted state), to skimp on strength training because you don't like it (it's good for you!), or because you fear it will make you "bulk up" (it won't), and so forth. The training prescribed here is probably different from what you're used to, but that's a good thing. I promise: This is the right way to train to maximize fat loss and get ready for your next training cycle.

LOW-VOLUME TRAINING PLANS

FOR CYCLISTS

4, 6 & 8 WEEKS

WEEK 1

Cycling Volume: 3:20   Total Training Volume: 4:00

MONDAY

Rest

TUESDAY
Power Intervals

10 minutes easy

12 x 10 seconds max effort in large gear (high resistance).
Spin 1 minute after each sprint.

10 minutes easy

WEDNESDAY
Strength Workout, *1 circuit*

EXERCISE	REPETITIONS
Step-up	10 per leg
Stick crunch	12
Chin-up	10
Single-leg squat	10 per leg
Side plank	30 seconds per side
Push-up	20 or to failure
Supine gluteal activation	10 per leg
L-over	6 per side
Inverted shoulder press	10
Eccentric heel dip	12 per leg

THURSDAY
Easy Ride

45 minutes easy

FRIDAY
Speed Intervals

10 minutes easy

8 x 30 seconds max effort at high cadence.
Spin 1 minute after each sprint.

10 minutes easy

SATURDAY
Strength Workout, *1 circuit*

EXERCISE	REPETITIONS
Step-up	10 per leg
Stick crunch	12
Chin-up	10
Single-leg squat	10 per leg
Side plank	30 seconds per side
Push-up	20 or to failure
Supine gluteal activation	10 per leg
L-over	6 per side
Inverted shoulder press	10
Eccentric heel dip	12 per leg

SUNDAY
Fat-Burning Ride

1 hour 30 minutes easy in fasted state

CYCLISTS · LOW VOLUME · WEEK 1

WEEK 2

Cycling Volume: 3:45   Total Training Volume: 4:25

MONDAY

Rest

TUESDAY
Hill Sprints

10 minutes easy

10 x 20 seconds max effort uphill.
Spin 1 minute after each sprint.

10 minutes easy

WEDNESDAY
Strength Workout, *1 circuit*

EXERCISE	REPETITIONS
Elevated reverse lunge	10 per leg
Stick crunch	12
Chin-up	10
Single-leg squat	10 per leg
Side plank	30 seconds per side
Push-up	20 or to failure
Gluteal-hamstring raise	10 per leg
L-over	6 per side
Inverted shoulder press	10
Eccentric heel dip	12 per leg

THURSDAY
Easy Ride

50 minutes easy

FRIDAY
Power Intervals

10 minutes easy

14 x 10 seconds max effort in large gear (high resistance).
Spin 1 minute after each sprint.

10 minutes easy

SATURDAY
Strength Workout, *1 circuit*

EXERCISE	REPETITIONS
Giant walking lunge	10 per leg
Stick crunch	12
Chin-up	10
Single-leg squat	10 per leg
Side plank	30 seconds per side
Push-up	20 or to failure
Supine gluteal activation	10 per leg
L-over	6 per side
Inverted shoulder press	10
Eccentric heel dip	12 per leg

SUNDAY
Fat-Burning Ride

1 hour 45 minutes easy in fasted state

WEEK 3

Cycling Volume: 4:05   Total Training Volume: 5:25

MONDAY

Rest

TUESDAY
Speed Intervals

10 minutes easy

10 x 30 seconds max effort at high cadence.
Spin 1 minute after each sprint.

10 minutes easy

WEDNESDAY
Strength Workout, *2 circuits*

EXERCISE	REPETITIONS
Elevated reverse lunge	10 per leg
Stick crunch	12
Chin-up	10
Single-leg squat	10 per leg
Side plank	30 seconds per side
Push-up	20 or to failure
Gluteal-hamstring raise	10 per leg
L-over	6 per side
One-arm dumbbell snatch	10
Eccentric heel dip	12 per leg

THURSDAY
Easy Ride

55 minutes easy

FRIDAY
Hill Sprints

10 minutes easy

12 x 20 seconds max effort uphill.
Spin 1 minute after each sprint.

10 minutes easy

SATURDAY
Strength Workout, *2 circuits*

EXERCISE	REPETITIONS
Giant walking lunge	10 per leg
Stick crunch	12
Chin-up	10
Push press	10 per leg
Side plank	30 seconds per side
Push-up	20 or to failure
Supine gluteal activation	10 per leg
L-over	6 per side
Inverted shoulder press	10
Eccentric heel dip	12 per leg

SUNDAY
Fat-Burning Ride

2 hours easy in fasted state

WEEK 4
Cycling Volume: 4:05   Total Training Volume: 5:25

MONDAY

Rest

TUESDAY
Power Intervals

10 minutes easy

14 x 10 seconds max effort in large gear (high resistance).
Spin 1 minute after each sprint.

10 minutes easy

WEDNESDAY
Strength Workout, *2 circuits*

EXERCISE	REPETITIONS
Elevated reverse lunge	10 per leg
Stick crunch	12
Chin-up	10
Single-leg squat	10 per leg
Side plank	30 seconds per side
Push-up	20 or to failure
Gluteal-hamstring raise	10 per leg
Suitcase deadlift	10 per side
One-arm dumbbell snatch	10
Eccentric heel dip	12 per leg

THURSDAY
Easy Ride

50 minutes easy

FRIDAY
Speed Intervals

10 minutes easy

12 x 30 seconds max effort at high cadence.
Spin 1 minute after each sprint.

10 minutes easy

SATURDAY
Strength Workout, *2 circuits*

EXERCISE	REPETITIONS
Giant walking lunge	10 per leg
Stick crunch	12
Chin-up	10
Push press	10 per leg
Side plank	30 seconds per side
Push-up	20 or to failure
Supine gluteal activation	10 per leg
Suitcase deadlift	10 per side
Inverted shoulder press	10
Eccentric heel dip	12 per leg

SUNDAY
Fat-Burning Ride

2 hours easy in fasted state

CYCLISTS · LOW VOLUME · WEEK 4

WEEK 5
Cycling Volume: 4:33   Total Training Volume: 6:13

MONDAY

Rest

TUESDAY
Hill Sprints

10 minutes easy

14 x 20 seconds max effort uphill.
Spin 1 minute after each sprint.

10 minutes easy

WEDNESDAY
Strength Workout, *3 circuits*

EXERCISE	REPETITIONS
Elevated reverse lunge	10 per leg
Stick crunch	12
Chin-up	10
Single-leg squat	10 per leg
Plank	30 seconds
Push-up	20 or to failure
Gluteal-hamstring raise	10 per leg
Suitcase deadlift	10 per side
One-arm dumbbell snatch	10
Eccentric heel dip	12 per leg

THURSDAY
Easy Ride

1 hour easy

FRIDAY
Power Intervals

10 minutes easy

16 x 10 seconds max effort in large gear (high resistance).
Spin 1 minute after each sprint.

10 minutes easy

SATURDAY
Strength Workout, *2 circuits*

EXERCISE	REPETITIONS
Giant walking lunge	10 per leg
Stick crunch	12
Chin-up	10
Push press	10 per leg
Plank	30 seconds
Push-up	20 or to failure
Supine gluteal activation	10 per leg
Suitcase deadlift	10 per side
Inverted shoulder press	10
Eccentric heel dip	12 per leg

SUNDAY
Fat-Burning Ride

2 hours 15 minutes easy

WEEK 6

Cycling Volume: 4:35   Total Training Volume: 6:35

MONDAY

Rest

TUESDAY
Speed Intervals

10 minutes easy

14 x 30 seconds max effort at high cadence.
Spin 1 minute after each sprint.

10 minutes easy

WEDNESDAY
Strength Workout, *3 circuits*

EXERCISE	REPETITIONS
Elevated reverse lunge	10 per leg
Stick crunch	12
Chin-up	10
Single-leg squat	10 per leg
Reverse plank	30 seconds
Push-up	20 or to failure
Split-stance dumbbell deadlift	10 per side
L-over	8 per side
One-arm dumbbell snatch	10
Eccentric heel dip	12 per leg

THURSDAY
Easy Ride

1 hour easy

FRIDAY
Hill Sprints

10 minutes easy

16 x 20 seconds max effort uphill.
Spin 1 minute after each sprint.

10 minutes easy

SATURDAY
Strength Workout, *3 circuits*

EXERCISE	REPETITIONS
Giant walking lunge	10 per leg
Stick crunch	12
Chin-up	10
Push press	10 per leg
Plank	30 seconds
Push-up	20 or to failure
Split-stance dumbbell deadlift	10 per side
L-over	8 per side
Inverted shoulder press	10
Eccentric heel dip	12 per leg

SUNDAY
Fat-Burning Ride

2 hours 15 minutes easy

WEEK 7

Cycling Volume: 4:52   Total Training Volume: 6:52

MONDAY

Rest

TUESDAY
Power Intervals

10 minutes easy

18 x 10 seconds max effort in large gear (high resistance).
Spin 1 minute after each sprint.

10 minutes easy

WEDNESDAY
Strength Workout, *3 circuits*

EXERCISE	REPETITIONS
Elevated reverse lunge	10 per leg
Stick crunch	12
Chin-up	10
Single-leg squat	10 per leg
Reverse plank	30 seconds
Push-up	20 or to failure
Split-stance dumbbell deadlift	10 per side
L-over	8 per side
One-arm dumbbell snatch	10
Eccentric heel dip	12 per leg

THURSDAY
Easy Ride

1 hour easy

FRIDAY
Speed Intervals

10 minutes easy

14 x 30 seconds max effort at high cadence.
Spin 1 minute after each sprint.

10 minutes easy

SATURDAY
Strength Workout, *3 circuits*

EXERCISE	REPETITIONS
Giant walking lunge	10 per leg
Stick crunch	12
Chin-up	10
Push press	10 per leg
Plank	30 seconds
Push-up	20 or to failure
Split-stance dumbbell deadlift	10 per side
L-over	8 per side
Inverted shoulder press	10
Eccentric heel dip	12 per leg

SUNDAY
Fat-Burning Ride

2 hours 30 minutes easy

WEEK 8
Cycling Volume: 4:57   Total Training Volume: 6:57

MONDAY

Rest

TUESDAY
Hill Sprints

10 minutes easy

18 x 20 seconds max effort uphill.
Spin 1 minute after each sprint.

10 minutes easy

WEDNESDAY
Strength Workout, *3 circuits*

EXERCISE	REPETITIONS
Elevated reverse lunge	10 per leg
Stick crunch	12
Chin-up	10
Single-leg squat	10 per leg
Reverse plank	30 seconds
Push-up	20 or to failure
Split-stance dumbbell deadlift	10 per side
L-over	8 per side
One-arm dumbbell snatch	10
Eccentric heel dip	12 per leg

THURSDAY
Easy Ride

1 hour easy

FRIDAY
Power Intervals

10 minutes easy

20 x 10 seconds max effort in large gear (high resistance).
Spin 1 minute after each sprint.

10 minutes easy

SATURDAY
Strength Workout, *3 circuits*

EXERCISE	REPETITIONS
Giant walking lunge	10 per leg
Stick crunch	12
Chin-up	10
Push press	10 per leg
Plank	30 seconds
Push-up	20 or to failure
Split-stance dumbbell deadlift	10 per side
L-over	8 per side
Inverted shoulder press	10
Eccentric heel dip	12 per leg

SUNDAY
Fat-Burning Ride

2 hours 30 minutes easy

CYCLISTS · LOW VOLUME · WEEK 8

HIGH-VOLUME
TRAINING PLANS
FOR CYCLISTS

4, 6 & 8 WEEKS

WEEK 1

Cycling Volume: 7:46   **Total Training Volume: 8:46**

MONDAY
Easy Ride

1 hour easy

Strength Workout, *1 circuit*

EXERCISE	REPETITIONS
Step-up	10 per leg
Stick crunch	12
Chin-up	10
Single-leg squat	10 per leg
Side plank	30 seconds per side
Push-up	20 or to failure
Supine gluteal activation	10 per leg
L-over	6 per side
Inverted shoulder press	10
Eccentric heel dip	12 per leg

TUESDAY
Power Intervals

20 minutes easy

12 x 10 seconds max effort in large gear (high resistance).
Spin 1 minute after each sprint.

20 minutes easy

WEDNESDAY
Easy Ride

1 hour easy

Strength Workout, *1 circuit*

EXERCISE	REPETITIONS
Step-up	10 per leg
Stick crunch	12
Chin-up	10
Single-leg squat	10 per leg
Side plank	30 seconds per side
Push-up	20 or to failure
Supine gluteal activation	10 per leg
L-over	6 per side
Inverted shoulder press	10
Eccentric heel dip	12 per leg

THURSDAY
Speed Intervals

20 minutes easy

8 x 30 seconds max effort at high cadence.
Spin 1 minute after each sprint.

20 minutes easy

FRIDAY
Easy Ride

1 hour easy

Strength Workout, *1 circuit*

EXERCISE	REPETITIONS
Step-up	10 per leg
Stick crunch	12
Chin-up	10
Single-leg squat	10 per leg
Side plank	30 seconds per side
Push-up	20 or to failure
Supine gluteal activation	10 per leg
L-over	6 per side
Inverted shoulder press	10
Eccentric heel dip	12 per leg

SATURDAY
Fat-Burning Ride

2 hours easy in fasted state

SUNDAY
Easy Ride

1 hour easy

WEEK 2
Cycling Volume: 8:20   Total Training Volume: 9:20

MONDAY
Easy Ride

1 hour easy

Strength Workout, *1 circuit*

EXERCISE	REPETITIONS
Elevated reverse lunge	10 per leg
Stick crunch	12
Chin-up	10
Single-leg squat	10 per leg
Side plank	30 seconds per side
Push-up	20 or to failure
Gluteal-hamstring raise	10 per leg
L-over	6 per side
Inverted shoulder press	10
Eccentric heel dip	12 per leg

TUESDAY
Hill Sprints

20 minutes easy

10 x 20 seconds max effort uphill.
Spin 1 minute after each sprint.

20 minutes easy

WEDNESDAY
Easy Ride

1 hour easy

Strength Workout, *1 circuit*

EXERCISE	REPETITIONS
Elevated reverse lunge	10 per leg
Stick crunch	12
Chin-up	10
Single-leg squat	10 per leg
Side plank	30 seconds per side
Push-up	20 or to failure
Gluteal-hamstring raise	10 per leg
L-over	6 per side
Inverted shoulder press	10
Eccentric heel dip	12 per leg

THURSDAY
Power Intervals

20 minutes easy

15 x 10 seconds max effort in large gear (high resistance).
Spin 1 minute after each sprint.

20 minutes easy

FRIDAY
Easy Ride

1 hour easy

Strength Workout, *1 circuit*

EXERCISE	REPETITIONS
Giant walking lunge	10 per leg
Stick crunch	12
Chin-up	10
Single-leg squat	10 per leg
Side plank	30 seconds per side
Push-up	20 or to failure
Supine gluteal activation	10 per leg
L-over	6 per side
Inverted shoulder press	10
Eccentric heel dip	12 per leg

SATURDAY
Fat-Burning Ride

2 hours 15 minutes easy in fasted state

SUNDAY
Easy Ride

1 hour 15 minutes easy

WEEK 3

Cycling Volume: 8:48   Total Training Volume: 10:48

MONDAY
Easy Ride

1 hour easy

Strength Workout, *2 circuits*

EXERCISE	REPETITIONS
Elevated reverse lunge	10 per leg
Stick crunch	12
Chin-up	10
Single-leg squat	10 per leg
Side plank	30 seconds per side
Push-up	20 or to failure
Gluteal-hamstring raise	10 per leg
L-over	6 per side
One-arm dumbbell snatch	10
Eccentric heel dip	12 per leg

TUESDAY
Speed Intervals

20 minutes easy
11 x 30 seconds max effort at high cadence. Spin 1 minute after each sprint.
20 minutes easy

WEDNESDAY
Easy Ride

1 hour 10 minutes easy

Strength Workout, *2 circuits*

EXERCISE	REPETITIONS
Elevated reverse lunge	10 per leg
Stick crunch	12
Chin-up	10
Single-leg squat	10 per leg
Side plank	30 seconds per side
Push-up	20 or to failure
Gluteal-hamstring raise	10 per leg
L-over	6 per side
One-arm dumbbell snatch	10
Eccentric heel dip	12 per leg

THURSDAY
Hill Sprints

20 minutes easy

13 x 20 seconds max effort uphill.
Spin 1 minute after each sprint.

20 minutes easy

FRIDAY
Easy Ride

1 hour easy

Strength Workout, *2 circuits*

EXERCISE	REPETITIONS
Giant walking lunge	10 per leg
Stick crunch	12
Chin-up	10
Push press	10 per leg
Side plank	30 seconds per side
Push-up	20 or to failure
Supine gluteal activation	10 per leg
L-over	6 per side
Inverted shoulder press	10
Eccentric heel dip	12 per leg

SATURDAY
Fat-Burning Ride

2 hours 30 minutes easy in fasted state

SUNDAY
Easy Ride

1 hour 15 minutes easy

WEEK 4
Cycling Volume: 8:00   Total Training Volume: 9:20

MONDAY

Rest

TUESDAY
Power Intervals

20 minutes easy

16 x 10 seconds max effort in large gear (high resistance).
Spin 1 minute after each sprint.

20 minutes easy

WEDNESDAY
Easy Ride

1 hour easy

Strength Workout, *2 circuits*

EXERCISE	REPETITIONS
Elevated reverse lunge	10 per leg
Stick crunch	12
Chin-up	10
Single-leg squat	10 per leg
Side plank	30 seconds per side
Push-up	20 or to failure
Gluteal-hamstring raise	10 per leg
Suitcase deadlift	10 per side
One-arm dumbbell snatch	10
Eccentric heel dip	12 per leg

THURSDAY
Speed Intervals

20 minutes easy

14 x 30 seconds max effort at high cadence.
Spin 1 minute after each sprint.

20 minutes easy

FRIDAY
Easy Ride

1 hour easy

Strength Workout, *2 circuits*

EXERCISE	REPETITIONS
Giant walking lunge	10 per leg
Stick crunch	12
Chin-up	10
Push press	10 per leg
Side plank	30 seconds per side
Push-up	20 or to failure
Supine gluteal activation	10 per leg
Suitcase deadlift	10 per side
Inverted shoulder press	10
Eccentric heel dip	12 per leg

SATURDAY
Fat-Burning Ride

2 hours 30 minutes easy in fasted state

SUNDAY
Easy Ride

1 hour 30 minutes easy

WEEK 5
Cycling Volume: 9:25   Total Training Volume: 12:05

MONDAY
Easy Ride

1 hour easy

Strength Workout, *3 circuits*

EXERCISE	REPETITIONS
Elevated reverse lunge	10 per leg
Stick crunch	12
Chin-up	10
Single-leg squat	10 per leg
Plank	30 seconds
Push-up	20 or to failure
Gluteal-hamstring raise	10 per leg
Suitcase deadlift	10 per side
One-arm dumbbell snatch	10
Eccentric heel dip	12 per leg

TUESDAY
Hill Sprints

20 minutes easy

16 x 20 seconds max effort uphill.
Spin 1 minute after each sprint.

20 minutes easy

WEDNESDAY
Easy Ride

1 hour 10 minutes easy

Strength Workout, *3 circuits*

EXERCISE	REPETITIONS
Elevated reverse lunge	10 per leg
Stick crunch	12
Chin-up	10
Single-leg squat	10 per leg
Plank	30 seconds
Push-up	20 or to failure
Gluteal-hamstring raise	10 per leg
Suitcase deadlift	10 per side
One-arm dumbbell snatch	10
Eccentric heel dip	12 per leg

THURSDAY
Power Intervals

20 minutes easy

18 x 10 seconds max effort in large gear (high resistance).
Spin 1 minute after each sprint.

20 minutes easy

FRIDAY
Easy Ride

1 hour easy

Strength Workout, *2 circuits*

EXERCISE	REPETITIONS
Giant walking lunge	10 per leg
Stick crunch	12
Chin-up	10
Push press	10 per leg
Plank	30 seconds
Push-up	20 or to failure
Supine gluteal activation	10 per leg
Suitcase deadlift	10 per side
Inverted shoulder press	10
Eccentric heel dip	12 per leg

SATURDAY
Fat-Burning Ride

2 hours 45 minutes easy

SUNDAY
Easy Ride

1 hour 30 minutes easy

WEEK 6
Cycling Volume: 9:33   Total Training Volume: 12:38

MONDAY
Easy Ride

1 hour easy

Strength Workout, *3 circuits*

EXERCISE	REPETITIONS
Elevated reverse lunge	10 per leg
Stick crunch	12
Chin-up	10
Single-leg squat	10 per leg
Reverse plank	30 seconds
Push-up	20 or to failure
Split-stance dumbbell deadlift	10 per side
L-over	8 per side
One-arm dumbbell snatch	10
Eccentric heel dip	12 per leg

TUESDAY
Speed Intervals

20 minutes easy

16 x 30 seconds max effort at high cadence.
Spin 1 minute after each sprint.

20 minutes easy

WEDNESDAY
Easy Ride

1 hour easy

Strength Workout, *3 circuits*

EXERCISE	REPETITIONS
Elevated reverse lunge	10 per leg
Stick crunch	12
Chin-up	10
Single-leg squat	10 per leg
Reverse plank	30 seconds
Push-up	20 or to failure
Split-stance dumbbell deadlift	10 per side
L-over	8 per side
One-arm dumbbell snatch	10
Eccentric heel dip	12 per leg

THURSDAY
Hill Sprints

20 minutes easy

18 x 20 seconds max effort uphill.
Spin 1 minute after each sprint.

20 minutes easy

FRIDAY
Easy Ride

1 hour easy

Strength Workout, *3 circuits*

EXERCISE	REPETITIONS
Giant walking lunge	10 per leg
Stick crunch	12
Chin-up	10
Push press	10 per leg
Plank	30 seconds
Push-up	20 or to failure
Split-stance dumbbell deadlift	10 per side
L-over	8 per side
Inverted shoulder press	10
Eccentric heel dip	12 per leg

SATURDAY
Fat-Burning Ride

2 hours 45 minutes easy

SUNDAY
Easy Ride

1 hour 45 minutes easy

WEEK 7

Cycling Volume: 9:52 **Total Training Volume: 12:52**

MONDAY
Easy Ride

1 hour easy

Strength Workout, *3 circuits*

EXERCISE	REPETITIONS
Elevated reverse lunge	10 per leg
Stick crunch	12
Chin-up	10
Single-leg squat	10 per leg
Reverse plank	30 seconds
Push-up	20 or to failure
Split-stance dumbbell deadlift	10 per side
L-over	8 per side
One-arm dumbbell snatch	10
Eccentric heel dip	12 per leg

TUESDAY
Power Intervals

20 minutes easy

20 x 10 seconds max effort in large gear (high resistance).
Spin 1 minute after each sprint.

20 minutes easy

WEDNESDAY
Easy Ride

1 hour easy

Strength Workout, *3 circuits*

EXERCISE	REPETITIONS
Elevated reverse lunge	10 per leg
Stick crunch	12
Chin-up	10
Single-leg squat	10 per leg
Reverse plank	30 seconds
Push-up	20 or to failure
Split-stance dumbbell deadlift	10 per side
L-over	8 per side
One-arm dumbbell snatch	10
Eccentric heel dip	12 per leg

THURSDAY
Speed Intervals

20 minutes easy

16 x 30 seconds max effort at high cadence.
Spin 1 minute after each sprint.

20 minutes easy

FRIDAY
Easy Ride

1 hour easy

Strength Workout, *3 circuits*

EXERCISE	REPETITIONS
Giant walking lunge	10 per leg
Stick crunch	12
Chin-up	10
Push press	10 per leg
Plank	30 seconds
Push-up	20 or to failure
Split-stance dumbbell deadlift	10 per side
L-over	8 per side
Inverted shoulder press	10
Eccentric heel dip	12 per leg

SATURDAY
Fat-Burning Ride

3 hours easy

SUNDAY
Easy Ride

1 hour 45 minutes easy

WEEK 8
Cycling Volume: 9:12   **Total Training Volume:** 11:12

MONDAY

Rest

TUESDAY
Hill Sprints

20 minutes easy

20 x 20 seconds max effort uphill.
Spin 1 minute after each sprint.

20 minutes easy

WEDNESDAY
Easy Ride

1 hour easy

Strength Workout, *3 circuits*

EXERCISE	REPETITIONS
Elevated reverse lunge	10 per leg
Stick crunch	12
Chin-up	10
Single-leg squat	10 per leg
Reverse plank	30 seconds
Push-up	20 or to failure
Split-stance dumbbell deadlift	10 per side
L-over	8 per side
One-arm dumbbell snatch	10
Eccentric heel dip	12 per leg

THURSDAY
Power Intervals

20 minutes easy

22 x 10 seconds max effort in large gear (high resistance).
Spin 1 minute after each sprint.

20 minutes easy

FRIDAY
Easy Ride

1 hour easy

Strength Workout, *3 circuits*

EXERCISE	REPETITIONS
Giant walking lunge	10 per leg
Stick crunch	12
Chin-up	10
Push press	10 per leg
Plank	30 seconds
Push-up	20 or to failure
Split-stance dumbbell deadlift	10 per side
L-over	8 per side
Inverted shoulder press	10
Eccentric heel dip	12 per leg

SATURDAY
Fat-Burning Ride

3 hours easy

SUNDAY
Easy Ride

2 hours easy

EIGHT

TRAINING PLANS
FOR RUNNERS

D on't start training for your next marathon or any other important race before you've completed a quick start. That entails following a structured training plan designed especially to help you
lose fat quickly and build foundational fitness for future racing.
Here is a collection of such training plans: four-, six-, and eight-week
low-volume plans and four-, six-, and eight-week high-volume plans.
The six-week plans are extended versions of the four-week plans and
the eight-week plans are extended versions of the four- and six-week
plans, so only two schedules are presented. If, for example, you choose
to follow the six-week high-volume plan, just complete the workouts
in the first six weeks of the high-volume schedule and then move on
to your race-focused training. Do a four-week quick start if you are
within 10 lbs. of your racing eight, a six-week quick start if you are 11
to 20 lbs. above your racing weight, and an eight-week quick start if
you are more than 20 lbs. above your racing weight.

The low-volume plans feature six workouts per week: four runs and two strength workouts. The high-volume plans feature six runs and three strength workouts. The low-volume plans start with just over 2 hours of running and 3.5 hours of total training in Week 1 and peak at slightly over 3 hours of running and approximately 6 hours of total training in Week 8. The high-volume plans start with just over 4 hours of running and nearly 6 hours of total training in Week 1 and peak at roughly 7 hours of running and just under 11 hours of total training in Week 8.

Don't expect any of these plans to be a perfect fit. You may need to shuffle some workouts around to accommodate your schedule and make other small changes in accordance with your individual needs. For example, if you're a highly competitive and experienced runner who normally runs twice every day, go ahead and add a second, daily easy run to the high-volume schedule. Avoid making drastic changes to the workouts prescribed in these plans, however. The training approach may be somewhat novel for you, but it is the best approach for runners seeking quick weight loss before the start of a new training cycle.

LOW-VOLUME TRAINING PLANS
FOR RUNNERS
4, 6 & 8 WEEKS

WEEK 1

Running Volume: 2:16   Total Training Volume: 3:30

MONDAY

Rest

TUESDAY
Hill Intervals

Run 15 minutes easy

4 x 30 seconds hard up steep hill.
Jog back down for recovery.

Run 15 minutes easy

WEDNESDAY
Strength Workout, *1 circuit*

EXERCISE	REPETITIONS
Giant walking lunge	10 per leg
Side plank	30 seconds per side
Chin-up	10
Step-up	10 per leg
Alternating single-leg reverse crunch	10 per leg
Push-up	20 or to failure
Balance ball leg curl	10 per leg
Reverse plank	30 seconds
Inverted shoulder press	10
Eccentric heel dip	10 per leg

THURSDAY
Easy Run + Hill Sprint

Run 40 minutes at slow pace

1 x 10-second sprint up steep hill.
Walk back down for recovery.

FRIDAY
Cycling Power Intervals

Ride 10 minutes easy

12 x 10-second max effort in a high gear (high resistance).
Spin 1 minute after each interval.

Ride 10 minutes easy

SATURDAY
Strength Workout, *1 circuit*

EXERCISE	REPETITIONS
Single-leg squat	10 per leg
Side plank	30 seconds per side
Chin-up	10
Step-up	10 per leg
Alternating single-leg reverse crunch	10 per leg
Push-up	20 or to failure
Balance ball leg curl	10 per leg
Reverse plank	30 seconds
Inverted shoulder press	10
Eccentric heel dip	10 per leg

SUNDAY
Fat-Burning Run

1 hour easy in a fasted state drinking water only

RUNNERS • LOW VOLUME • WEEK 1

WEEK 2
Running Volume: 2:18   Total Training Volume: 3:34

MONDAY

Rest

TUESDAY
Hill Intervals

Run 15 minutes easy

5 x 30 seconds hard up steep hill.
Jog back down for recovery.

Run 15 minutes easy

WEDNESDAY
Strength Workout, *1 circuit*

EXERCISE	REPETITIONS
Single-leg squat	10 per leg
Side plank	30 seconds per side
Chin-up	10
Step-up	10 per leg
Alternating single-leg reverse crunch	10 per leg
Push-up	20 or to failure
Gluteal-hamstring raise	10
Reverse plank	30 seconds
Inverted shoulder press	10
Eccentric heel dip	10 per leg

THURSDAY
Easy Run + Hill Sprints

40 minutes easy

2 x 10-second sprints up steep hill.
Walk back down for recovery.

FRIDAY
Cycling Power Intervals

Ride 10 minutes easy

13 x 10-second max effort in a high gear (high resistance).
Spin 1 minute after each interval.

Ride 10 minutes easy

SATURDAY
Strength Workout, *1 circuit*

EXERCISE	REPETITIONS
Single-leg squat	10 per leg
Side plank	30 seconds per side
Chin-up	10
Split squat jump	10 per leg
Alternating single-leg reverse crunch	10 per leg
Push-up	20 or to failure
Gluteal-hamstring raise	10
Reverse plank	30 seconds
Inverted shoulder press	10
Eccentric heel dip	10 per leg

SUNDAY
Fat-Burning Run

1 hour easy in a fasted state drinking water only

WEEK 3

Running Volume: 2:34   Total Training Volume: 4:28

MONDAY

Rest

TUESDAY
Hill Intervals

Run 15 minutes easy

6 x 30 seconds hard up steep hill.
Jog back down for recovery.

Run 15 minutes easy

WEDNESDAY
Strength Workout, *2 circuits*

EXERCISE	REPETITIONS
Single-leg squat	10 per leg
Side plank	30 seconds per side
Chin-up	10
Split squat jump	10 per leg
Alternating single-leg reverse crunch	10 per leg
Push-up	20 or to failure
Gluteal-hamstring raise	10
Reverse plank	30 seconds
Inverted shoulder press	10
Eccentric heel dip	10 per leg

THURSDAY
Easy Run + Hill Sprints

45 minutes easy

3 x 10-second sprints up steep hill.
Walk back down for recovery.

FRIDAY
Cycling Power Intervals

Ride 10 minutes easy

12 x 10-second max effort in a high gear (high resistance).
Spin 1 minute after each interval.

Ride 10 minutes easy

SATURDAY
Strength Workout, *2 circuits*

EXERCISE	REPETITIONS
Single-leg squat	10 per leg
Side plank	30 seconds per side
Chin-up	10
Split squat jump	10 per leg
Alternating single-leg reverse crunch	10 per leg
Push-up	20 or to failure
Gluteal-hamstring raise	10
Reverse plank	30 seconds
Inverted shoulder press	10
Eccentric heel dip	10 per leg

SUNDAY
Fat-Burning Run

1 hour 10 minutes easy in a fasted state drinking water only

WEEK 4
Running Volume: 2:36   Total Training Volume: 4:32

MONDAY
Rest

TUESDAY
Hill Intervals

Run 15 minutes easy

7 x 30 seconds hard up steep hill.
Jog back down for recovery.

Run 15 minutes easy

WEDNESDAY
Strength Workout, *2 circuits*

EXERCISE	REPETITIONS
Single-leg squat	10 per leg
Side plank	30 seconds per side
Chin-up	10
Split squat jump	10 per leg
Alternating single-leg reverse crunch	10 per leg
Half-kneel cable pull	12 per side
Gluteal-hamstring raise	10
Reverse plank	30 seconds
Inverted shoulder press	10
Eccentric heel dip	10 per leg

THURSDAY
Easy Run + Hill Sprints

45 minutes easy

4 x 10-second sprints up steep hill.
Walk back down for recovery.

FRIDAY
Cycling Power Intervals

Ride 10 minutes easy

15 x 10-second max effort in a high gear (high resistance).
Spin 1 minute after each interval.

Ride 10 minutes easy

SATURDAY
Strength Workout, *2 circuits*

EXERCISE	REPETITIONS
Single-leg squat	10 per leg
Side plank	30 seconds per side
Chin-up	10
Split squat jump	10 per leg
Alternating single-leg reverse crunch	10 per leg
Half-kneel cable pull	12 per side
Romanian deadlift	10
Reverse plank	30 seconds
Inverted shoulder press	10
Eccentric heel dip	10 per leg

SUNDAY
Fat-Burning Run

1 hour 10 minutes easy in a fasted state drinking water only

RUNNERS • LOW VOLUME • WEEK 4

WEEK 5
Running Volume: 2:52   Total Training Volume: 5:11

MONDAY

Rest

TUESDAY
Hill Intervals

Run 15 minutes easy

8 x 30 seconds hard up steep hill.
Jog back down for recovery.

Run 15 minutes easy

WEDNESDAY
Strength Workout, *3 circuits*

EXERCISE	REPETITIONS
Single-leg squat	10 per leg
Side plank	30 seconds per side
Chin-up	10
Split squat jump	10 per leg
Alternating single-leg reverse crunch	10 per leg
Half-kneel cable pull	12 per side
Romanian deadlift	10
Reverse plank	30 seconds
Inverted shoulder press	10
Eccentric heel dip	10 per leg

THURSDAY
Easy Run + Hill Sprints

50 minutes easy

5 x 10-second sprints up steep hill.
Walk back down for recovery.

FRIDAY
Cycling Power Intervals

Ride 10 minutes easy

16 x 10-second max effort in a high gear (high resistance).
Spin 1 minute after each interval.

Ride 10 minutes easy

SATURDAY
Strength Workout, *2 circuits*

EXERCISE	REPETITIONS
Single-leg squat	10 per leg
Side plank	30 seconds per side
Chin-up	10
Split squat jump	10 per leg
Alternating single-leg reverse crunch	10 per leg
Half-kneel cable pull	12 per side
Romanian deadlift	10
Reverse plank	30 seconds
Inverted shoulder press	10
Eccentric heel dip	10 per leg

SUNDAY
Fat-Burning Run

1 hour 20 minutes easy in a fasted state drinking water only

WEEK 6
Running Volume: 2:54   Total Training Volume: 5:34

MONDAY

Rest

TUESDAY
Hill Intervals

Run 15 minutes easy

9 x 30 seconds hard up steep hill.
Jog back down for recovery.

Run 15 minutes easy

WEDNESDAY
Strength Workout, *3 circuits*

EXERCISE	REPETITIONS
Single-leg squat	10 per leg
Side plank	30 seconds per side
Chin-up	10
Split squat jump	10 per leg
Alternating single-leg reverse crunch	10 per leg
Half-kneel cable pull	12 per side
Romanian deadlift	10
Reverse plank	30 seconds
Inverted shoulder press	10
X-band walk	12 steps each direction

THURSDAY
Easy Run + Hill Sprints

50 minutes easy

6 x 10-second sprints up steep hill.
Walk back down for recovery.

FRIDAY
Cycling Power Intervals

Ride 10 minutes easy

17 x 10-second max effort in a high gear (high resistance).
Spin 1 minute after each interval.

Ride 10 minutes easy

SATURDAY
Strength Workout, *3 circuits*

EXERCISE	REPETITIONS
Single-leg squat	10 per leg
L-over	8 per side
Chin-up	10
Split squat jump	10 per leg
Alternating single-leg reverse crunch	10 per leg
Half-kneel cable pull	12 per side
Romanian deadlift	10
Reverse plank	30 seconds
Inverted shoulder press	10
Balancing bend and reach	10 per leg

SUNDAY
Fat-Burning Run

1 hour 20 minutes easy in a fasted state drinking water only

RUNNERS • LOW VOLUME • WEEK 6

WEEK 7
Running Volume: 3:11   Total Training Volume: 5:52

MONDAY

Rest

TUESDAY
Hill Intervals

Run 15 minutes easy

10 x 30 seconds hard up steep hill.
Jog back down for recovery.

Run 15 minutes easy

WEDNESDAY
Strength Workout, *3 circuits*

EXERCISE	REPETITIONS
Single-leg squat	10 per leg
L-over	8 per side
Chin-up	10
Split squat jump	10 per leg
Alternating single-leg reverse crunch	10 per leg
Half-kneel cable pull	12 per side
Romanian deadlift	10
Stick crunch	20
Inverted shoulder press	10
X-band walk	12 steps each direction

THURSDAY
Easy Run + Hill Sprints

55 minutes easy

7 x 10-second sprints up steep hill.
Walk back down for recovery.

FRIDAY
Cycling Power Intervals

Ride 10 minutes easy

18 x 10-second max effort in a high gear (high resistance).
Spin 1 minute after each interval.

Ride 10 minutes easy

SATURDAY
Strength Workout, *3 circuits*

EXERCISE	REPETITIONS
Single-leg squat	10 per leg
L-over	8 per side
Chin-up	10
Split squat jump	10 per leg
Alternating single-leg reverse crunch	10 per leg
Half-kneel cable pull	12 per side
Romanian deadlift	10
Stick crunch	20
Bent-over cable shoulder lateral extension	10 per arm
Balancing bend and reach	10 per leg

SUNDAY
Fat-Burning Run

1 hour 30 minutes easy in a fasted state drinking water only

WEEK 8
Running Volume: 3:16   Total Training Volume: 5:57

MONDAY

Rest

TUESDAY
Hill Intervals

Run 15 minutes easy

10 x 30 seconds hard up steep hill.
Jog back down for recovery.

Run 15 minutes easy

WEDNESDAY
Strength Workout, *3 circuits*

EXERCISE	REPETITIONS
Split-stance deadlift	10 per leg
L-over	8 per side
Chin-up	10
Split squat jump	10 per leg
Alternating single-leg reverse crunch	10 per leg
Half-kneel cable pull	12 per side
Romanian deadlift	10
Stick crunch	20
Bent-over cable shoulder lateral extension	10 per arm
X-band walk	12 steps each direction

THURSDAY
Easy Run + Hill Sprints

1 hour easy

8 x 10-second sprints up steep hill.
Walk back down for recovery.

FRIDAY
Cycling Power Intervals

Ride 10 minutes easy

18 x 10-second max effort in a high gear (high resistance).
Spin 1 minute after each interval.

Ride 10 minutes easy

SATURDAY
Strength Workout, *3 circuits*

EXERCISE	REPETITIONS
Split-stance deadlift	10 per leg
L-over	8 per side
Chin-up	10
Split squat jump	10 per leg
Alternating single-leg reverse crunch	10 per leg
Half-kneel cable pull	12 per side
Romanian deadlift	10
Stick crunch	20
Bent-over cable shoulder lateral extension	10 per arm
Balancing bend and reach	10 per leg

SUNDAY
Fat-Burning Run

1 hour 30 minutes easy in a fasted state drinking water only

HIGH-VOLUME TRAINING PLANS
FOR RUNNERS

4, 6 & 8 WEEKS

WEEK 1
Running Volume: 4:16   Total Training Volume: 5:50

MONDAY
Easy Run

40 minutes easy

Strength Workout, *1 circuit*

EXERCISE	REPETITIONS
Giant walking lunge	10 per leg
Side plank	30 seconds per side
Chin-up	10
Step-up	10 per leg
Alternating single-leg reverse crunch	10 per leg
Push-up	20 or to failure
Balance ball leg curl	10 per leg
Reverse plank	30 seconds
Inverted shoulder press	10
Eccentric heel dip	10 per leg

TUESDAY
Hill Intervals

Run 15 minutes easy

4 x 30 seconds hard up steep hill.
Jog back down for recovery.

Run 15 minutes easy

WEDNESDAY
Easy Run

40 minutes easy

Strength Workout, *1 circuit*

EXERCISE	REPETITIONS
Giant walking lunge	10 per leg
Side plank	30 seconds per side
Chin-up	10
Step-up	10 per leg
Alternating single-leg reverse crunch	10 per leg
Push-up	20 or to failure
Balance ball leg curl	10 per leg
Reverse plank	30 seconds
Inverted shoulder press	10
Eccentric heel dip	10 per leg

THURSDAY
Easy Run + Sprint

Run 40 minutes easy

1 x 10-second sprint up steep hill.
Walk back down for recovery.

FRIDAY
Cycling Power Intervals

Ride 10 minutes easy

12 x 10-second max effort in a high gear (high resistance).
Spin 1 minute after each interval.

Ride 10 minutes easy

Strength Workout, *1 circuit*

EXERCISE	REPETITIONS
Single-leg squat	10 per leg
Side plank	30 seconds per side
Chin-up	10
Step-up	10 per leg
Alternating single-leg reverse crunch	10 per leg
Push-up	20 or to failure
Balance ball leg curl	10 per leg
Reverse plank	30 seconds
Inverted shoulder press	10
Eccentric heel dip	10 per leg

SATURDAY
Easy Run

40 minutes easy

SUNDAY
Fat-Burning Run

1 hour easy in a fasted state drinking water only

WEEK 2
Running Volume: 4:55   Total Training Volume: 6:31

MONDAY
Easy Run

45 minutes easy

Strength Workout, *1 circuit*

EXERCISE	REPETITIONS
Single-leg squat	10 per leg
Side plank	30 seconds per side
Chin-up	10
Step-up	10 per leg
Alternating single-leg reverse crunch	10 per leg
Push-up	20 or to failure
Gluteal-hamstring raise	10
Reverse plank	30 seconds
Inverted shoulder press	10
Eccentric heel dip	10 per leg

TUESDAY
Hill Intervals

Run 15 minutes easy

6 x 30 seconds hard up steep hill.
Jog back down for recovery.

Run 15 minutes easy

WEDNESDAY
Easy Run

45 minutes easy

Strength Workout, *1 circuit*

EXERCISE	REPETITIONS
Single-leg squat	10 per leg
Side plank	30 seconds per side
Chin-up	10
Step-up	10 per leg
Alternating single-leg reverse crunch	10 per leg
Push-up	20 or to failure
Gluteal-hamstring raise	10
Reverse plank	30 seconds
Inverted shoulder press	10
Eccentric heel dip	10 per leg

THURSDAY
Easy Run + Hill Sprints

45 minutes easy

4 x 10-second sprints up steep hill.
Walk back down for recovery.

FRIDAY
Cycling Power Intervals

Ride 10 minutes easy

14 x 10-second max effort in a high gear (high resistance).
Spin 1 minute after each interval.

Ride 10 minutes easy

Strength Workout, *1 circuit*

EXERCISE	REPETITIONS
Single-leg squat	10 per leg
Side plank	30 seconds per side
Chin-up	10
Split squat jump	10 per leg
Alternating single-leg reverse crunch	10 per leg
Push-up	20 or to failure
Gluteal-hamstring raise	10
Reverse plank	30 seconds
Inverted shoulder press	10
Eccentric heel dip	10 per leg

SATURDAY
Easy Run

45 minutes easy

SUNDAY
Fat-Burning Run

1 hour 15 minutes easy in a fasted state drinking water only

RUNNERS · HIGH VOLUME · WEEK 2

WEEK 3
Running Volume: 5:23   **Total Training Volume: 8:00**

MONDAY
Easy Run

50 minutes easy

Strength Workout, *2 circuits*

EXERCISE	REPETITIONS
Single-leg squat	10 per leg
Side plank	30 seconds per side
Chin-up	10
Split squat jump	10 per leg
Alternating single-leg reverse crunch	10 per leg
Push-up	20 or to failure
Gluteal-hamstring raise	10
Reverse plank	30 seconds
Inverted shoulder press	10
Eccentric heel dip	10 per leg

TUESDAY
Hill Intervals

Run 15 minutes easy

8 x 30 seconds hard up steep hill.

Jog back down for recovery.

Run 15 minutes easy

WEDNESDAY
Easy Run

45 minutes easy

Strength Workout, *2 circuits*

EXERCISE	REPETITIONS
Single-leg squat	10 per leg
Side plank	30 seconds per side
Chin-up	10
Split squat jump	10 per leg
Alternating single-leg reverse crunch	10 per leg
Push-up	20 or to failure
Gluteal-hamstring raise	10
Reverse plank	30 seconds
Inverted shoulder press	10
Eccentric heel dip	10 per leg

THURSDAY
Easy Run + Hill Sprints

45 minutes easy

6 x 10-second sprints up steep hill.
Walk back down for recovery.

FRIDAY
Cycling Power Intervals

Ride 10 minutes easy

15 x 10-second max effort in a high gear (high resistance).
Spin 1 minute after each interval.

Ride 10 minutes easy

RUNNERS · HIGH VOLUME · WEEK 3

Strength Workout, *2 circuits*

EXERCISE	REPETITIONS
Single-leg squat	10 per leg
Side plank	30 seconds per side
Chin-up	10
Split squat jump	10 per leg
Alternating single-leg reverse crunch	10 per leg
Push-up	20 or to failure
Gluteal-hamstring raise	10
Reverse plank	30 seconds
Inverted shoulder press	10
Eccentric heel dip	10 per leg

SATURDAY
Easy Run

50 minutes

SUNDAY
Fat-Burning Run

1 hour 30 minutes easy in a fasted state drinking water only

WEEK 4

Running Volume: 5:01   Total Training Volume: 7:20

MONDAY
Easy Run

30 minutes easy

Strength Workout, *1 circuit*

EXERCISE	REPETITIONS
Single-leg squat	10 per leg
Side plank	30 seconds per side
Chin-up	10
Split squat jump	10 per leg
Alternating single-leg reverse crunch	10 per leg
Half-kneel cable pull	12 per side
Gluteal-hamstring raise	10
Reverse plank	30 seconds
Inverted shoulder press	10
Eccentric heel dip	10 per leg

TUESDAY
Hill Intervals

Run 15 minutes easy

10 x 30 seconds hard up steep hill.
Jog back down for recovery.

Run 15 minutes easy

WEDNESDAY
Easy Run

30 minutes easy

Strength Workout, *2 circuits*

EXERCISE	REPETITIONS
Single-leg squat	10 per leg
Side plank	30 seconds per side
Chin-up	10
Split squat jump	10 per leg
Alternating single-leg reverse crunch	10 per leg
Half-kneel cable pull	12 per side
Gluteal-hamstring raise	10
Reverse plank	30 seconds
Inverted shoulder press	10
Eccentric heel dip	10 per leg

THURSDAY
Easy Run + Hill Sprints

45 minutes easy

8 x 10-second sprints up steep hill.
Walk back down for recovery.

FRIDAY
Cycling Power Intervals

Ride 10 minutes easy

16 x 10-second max effort in a high gear (high resistance).
Spin 1 minute after each interval.

Ride 10 minutes easy

Strength Workout, *2 circuits*

EXERCISE	REPETITIONS
Single-leg squat	10 per leg
Side plank	30 seconds per side
Chin-up	10
Split squat jump	10 per leg
Alternating single-leg reverse crunch	10 per leg
Half-kneel cable pull	12 per side
Romanian deadlift	10
Reverse plank	30 seconds
Inverted shoulder press	10
Eccentric heel dip	10 per leg

SATURDAY
Easy Run

45 minutes easy

SUNDAY
Fat-Burning Run

1 hour 45 minutes easy in a fasted state drinking water only

RUNNERS • HIGH VOLUME • WEEK 4

WEEK 5

Running Volume: 6:24   Total Training Volume: 9:44

MONDAY
Easy Run

55 minutes easy

Strength Workout, *3 circuits*

EXERCISE	REPETITIONS
Single-leg squat	10 per leg
Side plank	30 seconds per side
Chin-up	10
Split squat jump	10 per leg
Alternating single-leg reverse crunch	10 per leg
Half-kneel cable pull	12 per side
Romanian deadlift	10
Reverse plank	30 seconds
Inverted shoulder press	10
Eccentric heel dip	10 per leg

TUESDAY
Hill Intervals

Run 15 minutes easy

12 x 30 seconds hard up steep hill.
Jog back down for recovery.

Run 15 minutes easy

WEDNESDAY
Easy Run

55 minutes easy

Strength Workout, *3 circuits*

EXERCISE	REPETITIONS
Single-leg squat	10 per leg
Side plank	30 seconds per side
Chin-up	10
Split squat jump	10 per leg
Alternating single-leg reverse crunch	10 per leg
Half-kneel cable pull	12 per side
Romanian deadlift	10
Reverse plank	30 seconds
Inverted shoulder press	10
Eccentric heel dip	10 per leg

THURSDAY
Easy Run + Hill Sprints

50 minutes easy

10 x 10-second sprints up steep hill.
Walk back down for recovery.

FRIDAY
Cycling Power Intervals

Ride 10 minutes easy

17 x 10-second max effort in a high gear (high resistance).
Spin 1 minute after each interval.

Ride 10 minutes easy

Strength Workout, *2 circuits*

EXERCISE	REPETITIONS
Single-leg squat	10 per leg
Side plank	30 seconds per side
Chin-up	10
Split squat jump	10 per leg
Alternating single-leg reverse crunch	10 per leg
Half-kneel cable pull	12 per side
Romanian deadlift	10
Reverse plank	30 seconds
Inverted shoulder press	10
Eccentric heel dip	10 per leg

SATURDAY
Easy Run

55 minutes easy

SUNDAY
Fat-Burning Run

2 hours easy in a fasted state drinking water only

WEEK 6
Running Volume: 6:51   Total Training Volume: 10:32

MONDAY
Easy Run

1 hour easy

Strength Workout, *3 circuits*

EXERCISE	REPETITIONS
Single-leg squat	10 per leg
Side plank	30 seconds per side
Chin-up	10
Split squat jump	10 per leg
Alternating single-leg reverse crunch	10 per leg
Half-kneel cable pull	12 per side
Romanian deadlift	10
Reverse plank	30 seconds
Inverted shoulder press	10
X-band walk	12 steps each direction

TUESDAY
Hill Intervals

Run 15 minutes easy

14 x 30 seconds hard up steep hill.
Jog back down for recovery.

Run 15 minutes easy

WEDNESDAY
Easy Run

1 hour easy

Strength Workout, *3 circuits*

EXERCISE	REPETITIONS
Single-leg squat	10 per leg
Side plank	30 seconds per side
Chin-up	10
Split squat jump	10 per leg
Alternating single-leg reverse crunch	10 per leg
Half-kneel cable pull	12 per side
Romanian deadlift	10
Reverse plank	30 seconds
Inverted shoulder press	10
X-band walk	12 steps each direction

THURSDAY
Easy Run + Hill Sprints

1 hour easy

10 x 10-second sprints up steep hill.
Walk back down for recovery.

FRIDAY
Cycling Power Intervals

Ride 10 minutes easy

18 x 10-second max effort in a high gear (high resistance).
Spin 1 minute after each interval.

Ride 10 minutes easy

Strength Workout, *3 circuits*

EXERCISE	REPETITIONS
Single-leg squat	10 per leg
L-over	8 per side
Chin-up	10
Split squat jump	10 per leg
Alternating single-leg reverse crunch	10 per leg
Half-kneel cable pull	12 per side
Romanian deadlift	10
Reverse plank	30 seconds
Inverted shoulder press	10
Balancing bend and reach	10 per leg

SATURDAY
Easy Run

1 hour easy

SUNDAY
Fat-Burning Run

2 hours easy in a fasted state drinking water only

WEEK 7
Running Volume: 6:04   Total Training Volume: 9:06

MONDAY
Easy Run

30 minutes easy

Strength Workout, *1 circuit*

EXERCISE	REPETITIONS
Single-leg squat	10 per leg
L-over	8 per side
Chin-up	10
Split squat jump	10 per leg
Alternating single-leg reverse crunch	10 per leg
Half-kneel cable pull	12 per side
Romanian deadlift	10
Stick crunch	20
Inverted shoulder press	10
X-band walk	12 steps each direction

TUESDAY
Hill Intervals

Run 15 minutes easy
12 x 30 seconds hard up steep hill. Jog back down for recovery.
Run 15 minutes easy

WEDNESDAY
Easy Run

1 hour easy

Strength Workout, *3 circuits*

EXERCISE	REPETITIONS
Single-leg squat	10 per leg
L-over	8 per side
Chin-up	10
Split squat jump	10 per leg
Alternating single-leg reverse crunch	10 per leg
Half-kneel cable pull	12 per side
Romanian deadlift	10
Stick crunch	20
Inverted shoulder press	10
X-band walk	12 steps each direction

THURSDAY
Easy Run + Hill Sprints

1 hour easy

10 x 10-second sprints up steep hill.
Walk back down for recovery.

FRIDAY
Cycling Power Intervals

Ride 10 minutes easy

19 x 10-second max effort in a high gear (high resistance).
Spin 1 minute after each interval.

Ride 10 minutes easy

RUNNERS · HIGH VOLUME · WEEK 7

Strength Workout, *3 circuits*

EXERCISE	REPETITIONS
Single-leg squat	10 per leg
L-over	8 per side
Chin-up	10
Split squat jump	10 per leg
Alternating single-leg reverse crunch	10 per leg
Half-kneel cable pull	12 per side
Romanian deadlift	10
Stick crunch	20
Bent-over cable shoulder lateral extension	10 per arm
Balancing bend and reach	10 per leg

SATURDAY
Easy Run

1 hour easy

SUNDAY
Fat-Burning Run

1 hour 45 minutes easy in a fasted state drinking water only

WEEK 8
Running Volume: 7:09   Total Training Volume: 10:53

MONDAY
Easy Run

1 hour easy

Strength Workout, *3 circuits*

EXERCISE	REPETITIONS
Split-stance deadlift	10 per leg
L-over	8 per side
Chin-up	10
Split squat jump	10 per leg
Alternating single-leg reverse crunch	10 per leg
Half-kneel cable pull	12 per side
Romanian deadlift	10
Stick crunch	20
Bent-over cable shoulder lateral extension	10 per arm
X-band walk	12 steps each direction

TUESDAY
Hill Intervals

Run 15 minutes easy

16 x 30 seconds hard up steep hill.
Jog back down for recovery.

Run 15 minutes easy

WEDNESDAY
Easy Run

1 hour easy

Strength Workout, *3 circuits*

EXERCISE	REPETITIONS
Split-stance deadlift	10 per leg
L-over	8 per side
Chin-up	10
Split squat jump	10 per leg
Alternating single-leg reverse crunch	10 per leg
Half-kneel cable pull	12 per side
Romanian deadlift	10
Stick crunch	20
Bent-over cable shoulder lateral extension	10 per arm
X-band walk	12 steps each direction

THURSDAY
Easy Run + Hill Sprints

1 hour easy

10 x 10-second sprints up steep hill.
Walk back down for recovery.

FRIDAY
Cycling Power Intervals

Ride 10 minutes easy

20 x 10-second max effort in a high gear (high resistance).
Spin 1 minute after each interval.

Ride 10 minutes easy

Strength Workout, *3 circuits*

EXERCISE	REPETITIONS
Split-stance deadlift	10 per leg
L-over	8 per side
Chin-up	10
Split squat jump	10 per leg
Alternating single-leg reverse crunch	10 per leg
Half-kneel cable pull	12 per side
Romanian deadlift	10
Stick crunch	20
Bent-over cable shoulder lateral extension	10 per arm
Balancing bend and reach	10 per leg

SATURDAY
Easy Run

1 hour easy

SUNDAY
Fat-Burning Run

2 hours 15 minutes easy in a fasted state drinking water only

RUNNERS · HIGH VOLUME · WEEK 8

TRAINING PLANS
FOR TRIATHLETES

n this chapter I present a selection of quick start training plans
for triathletes. There is a set of low-volume plans, encompassing
four-, six-, and eight-week durations, and also a set of high-volume
plans, of matching durations. The six-week plans are extended versions of the four-week plans, and the eight-week plans are extended
versions of the four- and six-week plans, so only two schedules are
presented. Choose your volume level and quick start duration and follow the relevant schedule either to the midpoint, the six-week mark,
or all the way through. I recommend that you go with a four-week
quick start if you are within 10 lbs. of your racing weight, do a six-
week quick start if you are 11 to 20 lbs. above your racing weight, and
complete a full eight-week quick start if you are more than 20 lbs.
above your racing weight.

The low-volume plans feature seven workouts per week: two
swims, two ride-runs, a run, and two strength workouts. The

high-volume plans feature 12 workouts per week: three swims, three rides, three runs, and three strength workouts. The low-volume plans start with just over 3.5 hours of total training in Week 1 and peak at nearly 7 hours of total training in Week 8. The high-volume plans start with close to 8 hours of total training in Week 1 and peak at approximately 12.5 hours of total training in Week 8. Your training time will vary depending on your swimming pace. I estimated times based on 2 minutes per 100 meters or yards.

There's no such thing as a prefabricated training plan that perfectly fits the needs of athletes for whom it was not individually designed. So you may need to shuffle some workouts around to accommodate your schedule and make other small changes in accordance with your individual needs. For example, your habitual training frequency may fall between the seven workouts per week in the low-volume plans and the 12 in the high-volume plans. If this is the case, there's nothing wrong with tweaking either of the two plans to create a nine-workouts-per-week plan that's just right for you. Avoid making drastic changes to the workouts prescribed in these plans, however. The training approach may be somewhat novel for you, but it is the best training approach for triathletes seeking quick weight loss before the start of a new training cycle.

LOW-VOLUME TRAINING PLANS
FOR TRIATHLETES

4, 6 & 8 WEEKS

WEEK 1
Triathlon Volume: 3:04   Total Training Volume: 3:44

MONDAY
Strength Workout, *1 circuit*

EXERCISE	REPETITIONS
Single-leg squat	10 per leg
Stick crunch	20
Push-up	20 or to failure
Step-up	10 per leg
L-over	6 per side
Chin-up	10
Supine gluteal activation	10 per side
Side plank	30 seconds per side
Inverted shoulder press	12
Eccentric heel dip	10 per leg

TUESDAY
Interval Swim

200 warm-up
6 x 25 technique drills (rest 0:10)
6 x 25 kick with fins (rest 0:15)
6 x 25 sprint (rest 0:15)
6 x 25 pull with paddles (rest 0:10)
200 cool-down

WEDNESDAY
Bike + Run
Bike

30 minutes easy

Run (immediately after bike)

5 minutes easy

4 x 30 seconds hard uphill.
Jog down for recovery.

5 minutes easy

THURSDAY
Strength Workout, *1 circuit*

EXERCISE	REPETITIONS
Giant walking lunge	10 per leg
Stick crunch	20
Push-up	20 or to failure
Step-up	10 per leg
L-over	6 per side
Chin-up	10
Supine gluteal activation	10 per side
Side plank	30 seconds per side
Inverted shoulder press	12
Eccentric heel dip	10 per leg

FRIDAY
Endurance Swim

1,000 steady freestyle

SATURDAY
Bike Power Intervals

10 minutes easy

12 x 10 seconds max effort in large gear (high resistance).
Spin 1 minute after each sprint.

10 minutes easy

SUNDAY
Fat-Burning Run

1 hour easy in fasted state

1 x 10-second hill sprint

WEEK 2
Triathlon Volume: 3:36   Total Training Volume: 4:16

MONDAY
Strength Workout, *1 circuit*

EXERCISE	REPETITIONS
Giant walking lunge	10 per leg
Stick crunch	20
Push-up	20 or to failure
Step-up	10 per leg
L-over	6 per side
Chin-up	10
Supine gluteal activation	10 per side
Side plank	30 seconds per side
Inverted shoulder press	12
Balancing bend and reach	10 per leg

TUESDAY
Interval Swim

200 warm-up
6 x 25 technique drills (rest 0:10)
8 x 25 kick with fins (rest 0:15)
8 x 25 sprint (rest 0:15)
6 x 25 pull with paddles (rest 0:10)
200 cool-down

WEDNESDAY
Bike Speed Intervals + Run
Bike

10 minutes easy

8 x 30 seconds max effort at high cadence.
Spin 1 minute after each sprint.

10 minutes easy

Run (immediately after bike)

15 minutes easy

2 x 10-second hill sprints.
Walk back down for recovery.

THURSDAY
Strength Workout, *1 circuit*

EXERCISE	REPETITIONS
Giant walking lunge	10 per leg
Alternating single-leg reverse crunch	20
Push-up	20 or to failure
Step-up	10 per leg
L-over	6 per side
Chin-up	10
Supine gluteal activation	10 per side
Side plank	30 seconds per side
Inverted shoulder press	12
Balancing bend and reach	10 per leg

FRIDAY
Endurance Swim

1,200 steady freestyle

SATURDAY
Fat-Burning Bike

1 hour 30 minutes easy in fasted state

SUNDAY
Run Hill Intervals

10 minutes easy

5 x 30 seconds uphill.
Jog down for recovery.

10 minutes easy

WEEK 3
Triathlon Volume: 3:41   Total Training Volume: 5:01

MONDAY
Strength Workout, *2 circuits*

EXERCISE	REPETITIONS
Giant walking lunge	10 per leg
Stick crunch	20
Push-up	20 or to failure
Step-up	10 per leg
L-over	6 per side
Chin-up	10
Supine gluteal activation	10 per side
Side plank	30 seconds per side
Cable face pull	12
Balancing bend and reach	10 per leg

TUESDAY
Swim

200 warm-up
6 x 25 technique drills (rest 0:10)
8 x 25 kick with fins (rest 0:15)
10 x 25 sprint (rest 0:15)
8 x 25 pull with paddles (rest 0:10)
200 cool-down

WEDNESDAY
Bike + Run
Bike

30 minutes easy

Run (immediately after bike)

5 minutes easy

6 x 30 seconds hard uphill.
Jog down for recovery.

5 minutes easy

THURSDAY
Strength Workout, *2 circuits*

EXERCISE	REPETITIONS
Split squat deadlift	10 per leg
Stick crunch	20
Push-up	20 or to failure
Step-up	10 per leg
L-over	6 per side
Chin-up	10
Supine gluteal activation	10 per side
Side plank	30 seconds per side
Cable face pull	12
Balancing bend and reach	10 per leg

FRIDAY
Endurance Swim

1,400 steady freestyle

SATURDAY
Bike Hill Sprints

15 minutes easy

10 x 20 seconds max effort uphill.
Spin 1 minute after each sprint.

15 minutes easy

SUNDAY
Fat-Burning Run

1 hour 10 minutes easy in fasted state

3 x 10-second hill sprints.
Walk back down for recovery.

WEEK 4
Triathlon Volume: 4:03   Total Training Volume: 5:23

MONDAY
Strength Workout, *2 circuits*

EXERCISE	REPETITIONS
Split squat deadlift	10 per leg
Stick crunch	20
One-arm dumbbell snatch	10 per arm
Step-up	10 per leg
L-over	6 per side
Chin-up	10
Supine gluteal activation	10 per side
Side plank	30 seconds per side
Cable face pull	12
Balancing bend and reach	10 per leg

TUESDAY
Swim

200 warm-up
6 x 25 technique drills (rest 0:10)
8 x 25 kick with fins (rest 0:15)
10 x 25 sprint (rest 0:15)
6 x 50 pull with paddles (rest 0:10)
200 cool-down

WEDNESDAY
Bike Power Intervals + Run
Bike

10 minutes easy

14 x 10 seconds max effort in large gear (high resistance).
Spin 1 minute after each sprint.

10 minutes easy

Run (immediately after bike)

15 minutes easy

2 x 10-second hill sprints

THURSDAY
Strength Workout, *2 circuits*

EXERCISE	REPETITIONS
Split squat deadlift	10 per leg
Stick crunch	20
One-arm dumbbell snatch	10 per arm
Step-up	10 per leg
Reverse plank	30 seconds
Chin-up	10
Supine gluteal activation	10 per side
Side plank	30 seconds per side
Cable face pull	12
Balancing bend and reach	10 per leg

FRIDAY
Endurance Swim

1,200 steady freestyle

SATURDAY
Fat-Burning Bike

1 hour 45 minutes easy in fasted state

SUNDAY
Run Hill Intervals

10 minutes easy

7 x 30 seconds uphill.

Jog down for recovery.

10 minutes easy

WEEK 5
Triathlon Volume: 3:55   Total Training Volume: 5:35

MONDAY
Strength Workout, *3 circuits*

EXERCISE	REPETITIONS
Split squat deadlift	10 per leg
Stick crunch	20
One-arm dumbbell snatch	10 per arm
Elevated reverse lunge	10 per leg
L-over	6 per side
Chin-up	10
Supine gluteal activation	10 per side
Side plank	30 seconds per side
Cable face pull	12
Balancing bend and reach	10 per leg

TUESDAY
Swim

200 warm-up
6 x 25 technique drills (rest 0:10)
6 x 50 kick with fins (rest 0:15)
10 x 25 sprint (rest 0:15)
6 x 50 pull with paddles (rest 0:10)
200 cool-down

WEDNESDAY
Bike + Run

Bike

30 minutes easy

Run (immediately after bike)

5 minutes easy

8 x 30 seconds hard uphill.
Jog down for recovery.

5 minutes easy

THURSDAY
Strength Workout, *2 circuits*

EXERCISE	REPETITIONS
Split squat deadlift	10 per leg
Stick crunch	20
One-arm dumbbell snatch	10 per arm
Elevated reverse lunge	10 per leg
L-over	6 per side
Chin-up	10
Gluteal-hamstring raise	10
Side plank	30 seconds per side
Cable face pull	12
Balancing bend and reach	10 per leg

FRIDAY
Endurance Swim

1,600 steady freestyle

SATURDAY
Bike Speed Intervals

15 minutes easy

12 x 30 seconds max effort at high cadence.
Spin 1 minute after each sprint.

15 minutes easy

SUNDAY
Fat-Burning Run

1 hour 20 minutes easy in fasted state

5 x 10-second hill sprints.
Walk back down for recovery.

WEEK 6
Triathlon Volume: 4:34 Total Training Volume: 6:34

MONDAY
Strength Workout, *3 circuits*

EXERCISE	REPETITIONS
Split squat deadlift	10 per leg
Stick crunch	20
One-arm dumbbell snatch	10 per arm
Elevated reverse lunge	10 per leg
L-over	6 per side
Chin-up	10
Gluteal-hamstring raise	10
Side plank	30 seconds per side
Cable face pull	12
Split squat jump	20

TUESDAY
Swim

200 warm-up
6 x 25 technique drills (rest 0:10)
6 x 50 kick with fins (rest 0:15)
6 x 50 sprint (rest 0:20)
6 x 50 pull with paddles (rest 0:10)
200 cool-down

WEDNESDAY
Bike Hill Sprints + Run
Bike

10 minutes easy
12 x 10 seconds max effort in large gear (high resistance). Spin 1 minute after each sprint.
10 minutes easy

Run (immediately after bike)

15 minutes easy
6 x 10-second hill sprints

THURSDAY
Strength Workout, *3 circuits*

EXERCISE	REPETITIONS
Kettlebell squat swing	30 seconds
Stick crunch	20
One-arm dumbbell snatch	10 per arm
Elevated reverse lunge	10 per leg
Suitcase deadlift	6 per side
Chin-up	10
Gluteal-hamstring raise	10
Side plank	30 seconds per side
Cable face pull	12
Split squat jump	20

FRIDAY
Endurance Swim

1,800 steady freestyle

SATURDAY
Fat-Burning Bike

2 hours easy in fasted state

SUNDAY
Run Hill Intervals

10 minutes easy

9 x 30 seconds uphill.
Jog down for recovery.

10 minutes easy

WEEK 7
Triathlon Volume: 4:24   Total Training Volume: 6:24

MONDAY
Strength Workout, *3 circuits*

EXERCISE	REPETITIONS
Kettlebell squat swing	30 seconds
Stick crunch	20
One-arm dumbbell snatch	10 per arm
Elevated reverse lunge	10 per leg
Suitcase deadlift	6 per side
Chin-up	10
Gluteal-hamstring raise	10
Side plank	30 seconds per side
Push press	12
Split squat jump	20

TUESDAY
Swim

200 warm-up
6 x 25 technique drills (rest 0:10)
6 x 50 kick with fins (rest 0:15)
8 x 50 sprint (rest 0:20)
6 x 50 pull with paddles (rest 0:10)
200 cool-down

WEDNESDAY
Bike + Run
Bike

30 minutes easy

Run (immediately after bike)

5 minutes easy

10 x 30 seconds hard uphill.
Jog down for recovery.

5 minutes easy

THURSDAY
Strength Workout, *3 circuits*

EXERCISE	REPETITIONS
Kettlebell squat swing	30 seconds
Stick crunch	20
One-arm dumbbell snatch	10 per arm
Elevated reverse lunge	10 per leg
Suitcase deadlift	6 per side
Bent-over cable shoulder lateral extension	10 per arm
Gluteal-hamstrings raise	10
Side plank	30 seconds per side
Push press	12
Split squat jump	20

FRIDAY
Endurance Swim

2,000 steady freestyle

SATURDAY
Bike Power Intervals

15 minutes easy

16 x 10 seconds max effort in large gear (high resistance).
Spin 1 minute after each sprint.

15 minutes easy

SUNDAY
Fat-Burning Run

1 hour 30 minutes easy in fasted state

6 x 10-second hill sprints.
Walk back down for recovery.

WEEK 8
Triathlon Volume: 4:51   Total Training Volume: 6:51

MONDAY
Strength Workout, *3 circuits*

EXERCISE	REPETITIONS
Kettlebell squat swing	30 seconds
Stick crunch	20
One-arm dumbbell snatch	10 per arm
Elevated reverse lunge	10 per leg
Suitcase deadlift	6 per side
Bent-over cable shoulder lateral extension	10 per arm
Romanian deadlift	10
Side plank	30 seconds per side
Push press	12
Hip hike	20 per side

TUESDAY
Swim

200 warm-up
6 x 25 technique drills (rest 0:10)
6 x 50 kick with fins (rest 0:15)
6 x 25 sprint (rest 0:15)
6 x 50 sprint (rest 0:20)
6 x 50 pull with paddles (rest 0:10)
200 cool-down

WEDNESDAY
Bike Speed Intervals + Run
Bike

10 minutes easy

14 x 30 seconds max effort at high cadence.
Spin 1 minute after each sprint.

10 minutes easy

Run (immediately after bike)

15 minutes easy

6 x 10-second hill sprints

THURSDAY
Strength Workout, *3 circuits*

EXERCISE	REPETITIONS
Kettlebell squat swing	30 seconds
Stick crunch	20
Push press	10
Elevated reverse lunge	10 per leg
Suitcase deadlift	6 per side
Bent-over cable shoulder lateral extension	10 per arm
Romanian deadlift	10
Alternating single-leg reverse crunch	12
Push press	12
Hip hike	20 per side

FRIDAY
Endurance Swim

2,000 steady freestyle

SATURDAY
Fat-Burning Bike

2 hours easy in fasted state

SUNDAY
Run Hill Intervals

10 minutes easy

10 x 30 seconds uphill.

Jog down for recovery.

10 minutes easy

HIGH-VOLUME TRAINING PLANS

FOR TRIATHLETES

4, 6 & 8 WEEKS

WEEK 1
Triathlon Volume: 6:45   Total Training Volume: 7:45

MONDAY
Strength Workout, *1 circuit*

EXERCISE	REPETITIONS
Single-leg squat	10 per leg
Stick crunch	20
Push-up	20 or to failure
Step-up	10 per leg
L-over	6 per side
Chin-up	10
Supine gluteal activation	10 per side
Side plank	30 seconds per side
Inverted shoulder press	12
Eccentric heel dip	10 per leg

TUESDAY
Interval Swim

400 warm-up
8 x 25 technique drills (rest 0:10)
8 x 25 kick with fins (rest 0:15)
3 x 100 base (rest 0:10)
12 x 25 sprint (rest 0:15)
8 x 25 pull with paddles (rest 0:10)
400 cool-down

Bike Power Intervals

20 minutes easy

12 x 10 seconds max effort in large gear (high resistance).
Spin 1 minute after each sprint.

20 minutes easy

WEDNESDAY
Easy Run + Hill Sprints

45 minutes easy

2 x 10-second sprints uphill.
Walk back down for recovery.

Strength Workout, *1 circuit*

EXERCISE	REPETITIONS
Single-leg squat	10 per leg
Stick crunch	20
Push-up	20 or to failure
Step-up	10 per leg
L-over	6 per side
Chin-up	10
Supine gluteal activation	10 per side
Side plank	30 seconds per side
Inverted shoulder press	12
Eccentric heel dip	10 per leg

THURSDAY
Swim Pull Set

200 warm-up

8 x 25 technique drills (rest 0:10)

8 x 25 kick with fins (rest 0:15)

20 x 50 freestyle with paddles (0:05), base effort except every
4th 50 hard

8 x 25 sprint (rest 0:15)

200 cool-down

Bike Easy Ride

1 hour easy

FRIDAY
Run Hill Intervals

Run 15 minutes easy

4 x 30 seconds hard up steep hill.
Jog back down for recovery.

Run 15 minutes easy

Strength Workout, *1 circuit*

EXERCISE	REPETITIONS
Giant walking lunge	10 per leg
Stick crunch	20
Push-up	20 or to failure
Step-up	10 per leg
L-over	6 per side
Chin-up	10
Supine gluteal activation	10 per side
Side plank	30 seconds per side
Inverted shoulder press	12
Eccentric heel dip	10 per leg

SATURDAY
Fat-Burning Bike

2 hours easy in fasted state

Endurance Swim

2,000 yards moderate

SUNDAY
Easy Run + Hill Sprints

45 minutes easy

2 x 10-second sprints uphill.
Walk back down for recovery.

WEEK 2

Triathlon Volume: 7:50   Total Training Volume: 8:50

MONDAY
Strength Workout, *1 circuit*

EXERCISE	REPETITIONS
Giant walking lunge	10 per leg
Stick crunch	20
Push-up	20 or to failure
Step-up	10 per leg
L-over	6 per side
Chin-up	10
Supine gluteal activation	10 per side
Side plank	30 seconds per side
Inverted shoulder press	12
Balancing bend and reach	10 per leg

TUESDAY
Interval Swim

400 warm-up
8 x 25 technique drills (rest 0:10)
8 x 25 kick with fins (rest 0:15)
4 x 100 base (rest 0:10)
12 x 25 sprint (rest 0:15)
8 x 25 pull with paddles (rest 0:10)
400 cool-down

Bike Speed Intervals

20 minutes easy

8 x 30 seconds max effort at high cadence.
Spin 1 minute after each sprint.

20 minutes easy

WEDNESDAY
Easy Run + Hill Sprints

45 minutes easy

3 x 10-second sprints uphill.
Walk back down for recovery.

Strength Workout, *1 circuit*

EXERCISE	REPETITIONS
Giant walking lunge	10 per leg
Stick crunch	20
Push-up	20 or to failure
Step-up	10 per leg
L-over	6 per side
Chin-up	10
Supine gluteal activation	10 per side
Side plank	30 seconds per side
Inverted shoulder press	12
Balancing bend and reach	10 per leg

THURSDAY
Swim Pull Set

200 warm-up

8 x 25 technique drills (rest 0:10)

8 x 25 kick with fins (rest 0:15)

12 x 100 freestyle with paddles (0:10), base effort except every 3rd 100 hard

8 x 25 sprint (rest 0:15)

200 cool-down

Bike Easy Ride

1 hour easy

FRIDAY
Run Hill Intervals

Run 15 minutes easy

6 x 30 seconds hard up steep hill.
Jog back down for recovery.

Run 15 minutes easy

Strength Workout, *1 circuit*

EXERCISE	REPETITIONS
Giant walking lunge	10 per leg
Alternating single-leg reverse crunch	20
Push-up	20 or to failure
Step-up	10 per leg
L-over	6 per side
Chin-up	10
Supine gluteal activation	10 per side
Side plank	30 seconds per side
Inverted shoulder press	12
Balancing bend and reach	10 per leg

TRIATHLETES • HIGH VOLUME • WEEK 2

SATURDAY
Bike Hill Sprints

20 minutes easy

10 x 20 seconds max effort uphill.
Spin 1 minute after each sprint.

20 minutes easy

Endurance Swim

2,200 yards moderate

SUNDAY
Fat-Burning Run

1 hour 15 minutes easy in fasted state

WEEK 3
Triathlon Volume: 8:00   Total Training Volume: 10:00

MONDAY
Strength Workout, *2 circuits*

EXERCISE	REPETITIONS
Giant walking lunge	10 per leg
Stick crunch	20
Push-up	20 or to failure
Step-up	10 per leg
L-over	6 per side
Chin-up	10
Supine gluteal activation	10 per side
Side plank	30 seconds per side
Cable face pull	12
Balancing bend and reach	10 per leg

TUESDAY
Interval Swim

400 warm-up
8 x 25 technique drills (rest 0:10)
8 x 25 kick with fins (rest 0:15)
4 x 100 base (rest 0:10)
14 x 25 sprint (rest 0:15)
8 x 25 pull with paddles (rest 0:10)
400 cool-down

Bike Power Intervals

20 minutes easy

15 x 10 seconds max effort in large gear (high resistance).
Spin 1 minute after each sprint.

20 minutes easy

WEDNESDAY
Easy Run + Hill Sprints

45 minutes easy

4 x 10-second sprints uphill.
Walk back down for recovery.

Strength Workout, *2 circuits*

EXERCISE	REPETITIONS
Giant walking lunge	10 per leg
Stick crunch	20
Push-up	20 or to failure
Step-up	10 per leg
L-over	6 per side
Chin-up	10
Supine gluteal activation	10 per side
Side plank	30 seconds per side
Cable face pull	12
Balancing bend and reach	10 per leg

THURSDAY
Swim Pull Set

200 warm-up

8 x 25 technique drills (rest 0:10)

8 x 25 kick with fins (rest 0:15)

24 x 50 freestyle with paddles (0:05), base effort except every 4th 50 hard

8 x 25 sprint (rest 0:15)

200 cool-down

Bike Easy Ride

1 hour easy

FRIDAY
Run Hill Intervals

Run 15 minutes easy

8 x 30 seconds hard up steep hill.
Jog back down for recovery.

Run 15 minutes easy

Strength Workout, *2 circuits*

EXERCISE	REPETITIONS
Split squat deadlift	10 per leg
Stick crunch	20
Push-up	20 or to failure
Step-up	10 per leg
L-over	6 per side
Chin-up	10
Supine gluteal activation	10 per side
Side plank	30 seconds per side

| Cable face pull | 12 |
| Balancing bend and reach | 10 per leg |

SATURDAY
Fat-Burning Bike

2 hours 15 minutes easy in fasted state

Endurance Swim

2,200 yards moderate

SUNDAY
Easy Run + Hill Sprints

50 minutes easy

5 x 10-second sprints uphill.
Walk back down for recovery.

WEEK 4
Triathlon Volume: 8:16   Total Training Volume: 10:16

MONDAY
Strength Workout, *2 circuits*

EXERCISE	REPETITIONS
Split squat deadlift	10 per leg
Stick crunch	20
One-arm dumbbell snatch	10 per arm
Step-up	10 per leg
L-over	6 per side
Chin-up	10
Supine gluteal activation	10 per side
Side plank	30 seconds per side
Cable face pull	12
Balancing bend and reach	10 per leg

TUESDAY
Interval Swim

400 warm-up
8 x 25 technique drills (rest 0:10)
8 x 25 kick with fins (rest 0:15)
4 x 100 base (rest 0:10)
16 x 25 sprint (rest 0:15)
8 x 25 pull with paddles (rest 0:10)
400 cool-down

Bike Speed Intervals

20 minutes easy

11 x 30 seconds max effort at high cadence.
Spin 1 minute after each sprint.

20 minutes easy

WEDNESDAY
Easy Run + Hill Sprints

45 minutes easy

6 x 10-second sprints uphill.
Walk back down for recovery.

Strength Workout, *2 circuits*

EXERCISE	REPETITIONS
Split squat deadlift	10 per leg
Stick crunch	20
One-arm dumbbell snatch	10 per arm
Step-up	10 per leg
L-over	6 per side
Chin-up	10
Supine gluteal activation	10 per side
Side plank	30 seconds per side
Cable face pull	12
Balancing bend and reach	10 per leg

THURSDAY
Swim Pull Set

200 warm-up

8 x 25 technique drills (rest 0:10)

8 x 25 kick with fins (rest 0:15)

15 x 100 freestyle with paddles (0:10), base effort except every
3rd 100 hard

8 x 25 sprint (rest 0:15)

200 cool-down

Bike Easy Ride

1 hour easy

FRIDAY
Run Hill Intervals

Run 15 minutes easy

10 x 30 seconds hard up steep hill.
Jog back down for recovery.

Run 15 minutes easy

Strength Workout, *2 circuits*

EXERCISE	REPETITIONS
Split squat deadlift	10 per leg
Stick crunch	20
One-arm dumbbell snatch	10 per arm
Step-up	10 per leg
Reverse plank	30 seconds
Chin-up	10
Supine gluteal activation	10 per side

Side plank	30 seconds per side
Cable face pull	12
Balancing bend and reach	10 per leg

SATURDAY
Bike Hill Sprints

20 minutes easy

13 x 20 seconds max effort uphill.
Spin 1 minute after each sprint.

20 minutes easy

Endurance Swim

2,400 yards moderate

SUNDAY
Fat-Burning Run

1 hour 30 minutes easy in fasted state

TRIATHLETES · HIGH VOLUME · WEEK 4

WEEK 5
Triathlon Volume: 9:17   Total Training Volume: 11:57

MONDAY
Strength Workout, *3 circuits*

EXERCISE	REPETITIONS
Split squat deadlift	10 per leg
Stick crunch	20
One-arm dumbbell snatch	10 per arm
Elevated reverse lunge	10 per leg
L-over	6 per side
Chin-up	10
Supine gluteal activation	10 per side
Side plank	30 seconds per side
Cable face pull	12
Balancing bend and reach	10 per leg

TUESDAY
Interval Swim

400 warm-up
8 x 25 technique drills (rest 0:10)
8 x 25 kick with fins (rest 0:15)
4 x 100 base (rest 0:10)
8 x 50 sprint (rest 0:20)
8 x 25 pull with paddles (rest 0:10)
400 cool-down

Bike Speed Intervals

20 minutes easy

14 x 30 seconds max effort at high cadence.
Spin 1 minute after each sprint.

20 minutes easy

WEDNESDAY
Easy Run + Hill Sprints

45 minutes easy

7 x 10-second sprints uphill.
Walk back down for recovery.

Strength Workout, *3 circuits*

EXERCISE	REPETITIONS
Split squat deadlift	10 per leg
Stick crunch	20
One-arm dumbbell snatch	10 per arm
Elevated reverse lunge	10 per leg
L-over	6 per side
Chin-up	10
Supine gluteal activation	10 per side
Side plank	30 seconds per side
Cable face pull	12
Balancing bend and reach	10 per leg

THURSDAY
Swim Pull Set

200 warm-up

8 x 25 technique drills (rest 0:10)

8 x 25 kick with fins (rest 0:15)

28 x 50 freestyle with paddles (0:05), base effort except every
4th 50 hard

8 x 25 sprint (rest 0:15)

200 cool-down

Bike Easy Ride

1 hour easy

FRIDAY
Run Hill Intervals

Run 15 minutes easy

12 x 30 seconds hard up steep hill.
Jog back down for recovery.

Run 15 minutes easy

Strength Workout, *2 circuits*

EXERCISE	REPETITIONS
Split squat deadlift	10 per leg
Stick crunch	20
One-arm dumbbell snatch	10 per arm
Elevated reverse lunge	10 per leg
L-over	6 per side
Chin-up	10
Gluteal-hamstrings raise	10

Side plank	30 seconds per side
Cable face pull	12
Balancing bend and reach	10 per leg

SATURDAY
Fat-Burning Bike

2 hours 30 minutes easy in fasted state

Endurance Swim

2,200 yards moderate

SUNDAY
Easy Run + Hill Sprints

55 minutes easy

8 x 10-second sprints uphill.
Walk back down for recovery.

WEEK 6
Triathlon Volume: 8:06   Total Training Volume: 11:06

MONDAY
Strength Workout, *3 circuits*

EXERCISE	REPETITIONS
Split squat deadlift	10 per leg
Stick crunch	20
One-arm dumbbell snatch	10 per arm
Elevated reverse lunge	10 per leg
L-over	6 per side
Chin-up	10
Gluteal-hamstring raise	10
Side plank	30 seconds per side
Cable face pull	12
Split squat jump	20

TUESDAY
Interval Swim

400 warm-up
8 x 25 technique drills (rest 0:10)
8 x 25 kick with fins (rest 0:15)
4 x 100 base (rest 0:10)
10 x 50 sprint (rest 0:20)
8 x 25 pull with paddles (rest 0:10)
400 cool-down

Bike Hill Sprints

20 minutes easy

16 x 20 seconds max effort uphill.
Spin 1 minute after each sprint.

20 minutes easy

WEDNESDAY
Easy Run + Hill Sprints

45 minutes easy

9 x 10-second sprints uphill.
Walk back down for recovery.

Strength Workout, *3 circuits*

EXERCISE	REPETITIONS
Split squat deadlift	10 per leg
Stick crunch	20
One-arm dumbbell snatch	10 per arm
Elevated reverse lunge	10 per leg
L-over	6 per side
Chin-up	10
Gluteal-hamstring raise	10
Side plank	30 seconds per side
Cable face pull	12
Split squat jump	20

TRIATHLETES · HIGH VOLUME · WEEK 6

THURSDAY
Swim Pull Set

200 warm-up

8 x 25 technique drills (rest 0:10)

8 x 25 kick with fins (rest 0:15)

15 x 100 freestyle with paddles (0:10), base effort except every 3rd 100 hard

8 x 25 sprint (rest 0:15)

200 cool-down

Bike Easy Ride

1 hour easy

FRIDAY
Run Hill Intervals

Run 15 minutes easy

14 x 30 seconds hard up steep hill.
Jog back down for recovery.

Run 15 minutes easy

Strength Workout, *3 circuits*

EXERCISE	REPETITIONS
Kettlebell squat swing	30 seconds
Stick crunch	20
One-arm dumbbell snatch	10 per arm
Elevated reverse lunge	10 per leg
Suitcase deadlift	6 per side
Chin-up	10
Gluteal-hamstring raise	10

Side plank	30 seconds per side
Cable face pull	12
Split squat jump	20

SATURDAY
Bike Power Intervals

20 minutes easy

18 x 10 seconds max effort in large gear (high resistance).
Spin 1 minute after each sprint.

20 minutes easy

Endurance Swim

2,400 yards moderate

SUNDAY
Fat-Burning Run

1 hour 45 minutes easy in fasted state

WEEK 7
Triathlon Volume: 9:59   Total Training Volume: 12:59

MONDAY
Strength Workout, *3 circuits*

EXERCISE	REPETITIONS
Kettlebell squat swing	30 seconds
Stick crunch	20
One-arm dumbbell snatch	10 per arm
Elevated reverse lunge	10 per leg
Suitcase deadlift	6 per side
Chin-up	10
Gluteal-hamstring raise	10
Side plank	30 seconds per side
Push press	12
Split squat jump	20

TUESDAY
Interval Swim

400 warm-up
8 x 25 technique drills (rest 0:10)
8 x 25 kick with fins (rest 0:15)
4 x 100 base (rest 0:10)
12 x 50 sprint (rest 0:20)
8 x 25 pull with paddles (rest 0:10)
400 cool-down

Bike Speed Intervals

20 minutes easy

16 x 30 seconds max effort at high cadence.
Spin 1 minute after each sprint.

20 minutes easy

WEDNESDAY
Easy Run + Hill Sprints

45 minutes easy

10 x 10-second sprints uphill.
Walk back down for recovery.

Strength Workout, *3 circuits*

EXERCISE	REPETITIONS
Kettlebell squat swing	30 seconds
Stick crunch	20
One-arm dumbbell snatch	10 per arm
Elevated reverse lunge	10 per leg
Suitcase deadlift	6 per side
Chin-up	10
Gluteal-hamstring raise	10
Side plank	30 seconds per side
Push press	12
Split squat jump	20

TRIATHLETES · HIGH VOLUME · WEEK 7

THURSDAY
Swim Pull Set

200 warm-up

8 x 25 technique drills (rest 0:10)

8 x 25 kick with fins (rest 0:15)

28 x 50 freestyle with paddles (0:05), base effort except every 4th 50 hard

8 x 25 sprint (rest 0:15)

200 cool-down

Bike Easy Ride

1 hour easy

FRIDAY
Run Hill Intervals

Run 15 minutes easy

12 x 30 seconds hard up steep hill.
Jog back down for recovery.

Run 15 minutes easy

Strength Workout, *3 circuits*

EXERCISE	REPETITIONS
Kettlebell squat swing	30 seconds
Stick crunch	20
One-arm dumbbell snatch	10 per arm
Elevated reverse lunge	10 per leg
Suitcase deadlift	6 per side
Bent-over cable shoulder lateral extension	10 per arm
Gluteal-hamstring raise	10

Side plank	30 seconds per side
Push press	12
Split squat jump	20

SATURDAY
Fat-Burning Bike

2 hours 30 minutes easy in fasted state

Endurance Swim

2,500 yards moderate

SUNDAY
Easy Run + Hill Sprints

1 hour easy

10 x 10-second sprints uphill.
Walk back down for recovery.

WEEK 8
Triathlon Volume: 9:34   Total Training Volume: 12:34

MONDAY
Strength Workout, *3 circuits*

EXERCISE	REPETITIONS
Kettlebell squat swing	30 seconds
Stick crunch	20
One-arm dumbbell snatch	10 per arm
Elevated reverse lunge	10 per leg
Suitcase deadlift	6 per side
Bent-over cable shoulder lateral extension	10 per arm
Romanian deadlift	10
Side plank	30 seconds per side
Push press	12
Hip hike	20 per side

TUESDAY
Interval Swim

400 warm-up
8 x 25 technique drills (rest 0:10)
8 x 25 kick with fins (rest 0:15)
4 x 100 base (rest 0:10)
8 x 25 sprint (rest 0:15)
8 x 50 sprint (rest 0:20)
8 x 25 pull with paddles (rest 0:10)
400 cool-down

Bike Hill Sprints

20 minutes easy

18 x 20 seconds max effort uphill.
Spin 1 minute after each sprint.

20 minutes easy

WEDNESDAY
Easy Run + Hill Sprints

45 minutes easy

10 x 10-second sprints uphill.
Walk back down for recovery.

Strength Workout, *3 circuits*

EXERCISE	REPETITIONS
Kettlebell squat swing	30 seconds
Stick crunch	20
One-arm dumbbell snatch	10 per arm
Elevated reverse lunge	10 per leg
Suitcase deadlift	6 per side
Bent-over cable shoulder lateral extension	10 per arm
Romanian deadlift	10
Side plank	30 seconds per side
Push press	12
Hip hike	20 per side

THURSDAY
Swim Pull Set

200 warm-up

8 x 25 technique drills (rest 0:10)

8 x 25 kick with fins (rest 0:15)

15 x 100 freestyle with paddles (0:10), base effort except every 3rd 100 hard

8 x 25 sprint (rest 0:15)

200 cool-down

Bike Easy Ride

1 hour easy

FRIDAY
Run Hill Intervals

Run 15 minutes easy

16 x 30 seconds hard up steep hill.
Jog back down for recovery.

Run 15 minutes easy

Strength Workout, *3 circuits*

EXERCISE	REPETITIONS
Kettlebell squat swing	30 seconds
Stick crunch	20
Push press	10
Elevated reverse lunge	10 per leg
Suitcase deadlift	6 per side
Bent-over cable shoulder lateral extension	10 per arm
Romanian deadlift	10

Alternating single-leg reverse crunch	12
Push press	12
Hip hike	20 per side

SATURDAY
Bike Power Intervals

20 minutes easy

20 x 10 seconds max effort in large gear (high resistance).
Spin 1 minute after each sprint.

20 minutes easy

Endurance Swim

2,500 yards moderate

SUNDAY
Fat-Burning Run

2 hours easy in fasted state

PUTTING IT ALL
TOGETHER

ndurance performance is a puzzle of many pieces. The attainment of optimal racing weight is one of those pieces. All else being equal, you will race better if you identify and actively work toward your personal racing weight.

Except for the few endurance athletes who always find themselves at or very close to their racing weight, the pursuit of racing weight is best approached as a two-step process. This book has focused on the first step: a four- to eight-week quick start comprising nutrition and training practices designed to yield rapid fat loss, while also laying the groundwork for a period of race-focused training to immediately follow. Step two is to follow the Racing Weight system while pursuing peak race fitness within a race-focused training cycle. Although based on the same underlying principles as the quick start protocol, the nutrition and training practices in the Racing Weight system are designed to maximize fitness increase through gradual, steady fat loss. Whether a single quick start and Racing Weight cycle will suffice to take you all the way to your racing weight will depend largely on how far you are above your racing weight. All you have to do to reach your racing weight eventually is to continue repeating this two-step process.

The quick start itself encompasses a few steps. We have looked at these steps individually in the preceding chapters. Here I'd like to bring them all together in a way that makes it easy for you to plan and execute your own quick start. The specific steps are:

1. Calculate your racing weight.

2. Select a target daily calorie deficit and quick start duration.

3. Choose a training plan and adjust it to better fit your schedule, fitness level, and goals.

4. Make sure you hit your daily calorie and protein targets.

Let's walk through this entire process so you have an example of how it all works, from quick start to finish. This will give you a clear picture of how the plan comes together. Rather than use a hypothetical athlete in this example, I will instead use a real athlete, who happens to be my younger brother, Sean.

SEAN'S QUICK START

At the time of this writing, Sean is 38 years old and an experienced recreational competitive runner. He's run several half marathons and a few marathons, with personal best times of 1:21 and 3:03 at the respective distances. These are pretty good times for a runner of any size, but are exceptionally good for a Clydesdale athlete who stands 6 feet 3 inches tall and weighs about 210 lbs. when he's not training seriously. Sean has always carried a bit of a belly, even when he has gotten his weight down to the low 190s before a marathon. On this basis alone he feels that he has not yet attained his ideal racing

> **▶ MODIFY VOLUME AND INTENSITY IN YOUR QUICK START TRAINING TO BE APPROPRIATE FOR YOUR NEEDS.**

weight. Thus, his quick start must begin with the calculation of an estimated racing weight.

STEP 1. CALCULATE ESTIMATED RACING WEIGHT

Sean currently weighs 206 lbs. and has a body composition of 19 percent fat. The racing weight body-fat range for men between the ages of 30 and 39 years is 5 to 12 percent. Following the guidelines presented in Chapter 1, Sean will set an initial goal of reducing his body fat to 12 percent. His chief reasons for not aiming lower are that historically he has had difficulty losing body fat, and he does not intend to train at the maximal level likely required to get his body fat down toward the low end of the ideal range for his age bracket.

To calculate his estimated racing weight, Sean must first calculate his body-fat mass, which is his current weight multiplied by his current body-fat percentage: 206×0.19, or approximately 39 lbs. Next, Sean must calculate his current lean body mass, which is simply his current weight minus his body-fat mass: $206 - 39$, or 167 lbs. Sean's estimated racing weight will equal his current lean body mass divided by his goal lean body mass percentage expressed in decimal form. Remember, goal lean body mass percentage is simply 1.0 – goal body fat percentage, or in this case $1.0 - 0.12 = 0.88$. So Sean's estimated racing weight is $167 \div 0.88$, or 190 lbs.

STEP 2. CHOOSE A QUICK START PLAN DURATION AND DAILY CALORIE DEFICIT

The difference between current weight and goal weight is the basis on which a quick start plan duration and daily caloric deficit are chosen. The farther you have to go, the longer your quick start and the larger your daily calorie deficit should be. Sean is currently 16 pounds above his racing weight. As you have seen, I recommend that those who are

11 to 20 pounds above their racing weight plan a six-week quick start and aim for a daily calorie deficit of 400 calories.

My recommendations for choosing a quick start format from among the three quick start options (four weeks with a 300-calorie-per-day deficit, six weeks with a 400-calorie-per-day deficit, and eight weeks with a 500-calorie-per-day deficit) based on your current weight relative to your ideal racing weight are only recommendations, not hard-and-fast laws. If, for example, you are more than 20 pounds above your racing weight and you prefer not to do the eight-week quick start that I recommend for those who exceed their racing weight by this amount, perhaps simply because you don't have time to squeeze it in along with a full training cycle before your next important race, you certainly don't have to. Just remember that the four-week plan is designed to yield roughly 4.5 pounds of weight loss, the six week plan to yield an eight-pound drop, give or take, and the eight-week plan to move you roughly 12 pounds closer to your racing weight, and make your selection based on these intended outcomes, if not strictly according to my recommendations.

You may also mix and match durations and calorie deficits. For example, if you don't have time for an eight-week quick start but you need and wish to lose more body fat than you would lose with the 300-calories-per-day deficit paired with the four week plan in this book, go ahead and combine a four-week quick start duration with a 500-calories-per-day deficit. I advise that you do not go outside the four- to eight-week duration parameters, however. Less than four weeks is not long enough to produce meaningful results. More than eight weeks will test the limits of your will power and take you away from race-focused training, and the fitness that comes with it, longer than you want. I also recommend that you stay within the range of 300 to 500 calories for your daily calorie deficit. Anything smaller than 300 calories will yield slower weight loss than you want, and anything above 500 calories is likely to sabotage your training by leaving your muscles chronically underfueled. But you don't have to adopt the specific calorie deficit I recommend based on the amount of weight loss you seek.

Sean will go by the book, though.

STEP 3. CHOOSE A TRAINING PLAN

Before you define your calorie intake target it is necessary to first choose a quick start training plan, because your training will obviously be a factor in your daily energy expenditure, which in turn is a factor in your daily calorie intake needs. In Sean's case, the low-volume running plan is most similar to his current training. Because he wants to run more often than four times per week, Sean will add a 20-minute easy warm-up run before each strength workout for an extra 40 minutes of running each week. This type of modification is something I encourage. Your quick start training must stay true to the core precepts embodied in the plans I've created, but it must also be appropriate to your needs in volume and intensity. Adding long tempo runs that make your diet impossible to maintain would be a poor choice. It's unlikely that any of the ready-made plans presented in Chapters 7–9 will be a perfect fit for you right out of the box.

STEP 4. CALCULATE DAILY CALORIE AND PROTEIN INTAKE TARGETS

Now Sean needs to determine how many calories he will aim to eat each day. This number will be the difference between his calculated daily calorie expenditure and his target energy deficit of 400 calories. His daily calorie expenditure will be the sum of the calories he burns in training over the first week of his quick start, the calories burned while sleeping (BMR), and the calories burned during nonexericse activity. He will get this total by following the instructions for counting calories (see Chapter 5).

To complete the job of calculating Sean's total daily calorie expenditure during the quick start, we refer to the training plan he has chosen to follow: the low-volume running plan with 40 minutes of additional easy running each week. With this in front of him, he can go back to racingweight.com and calculate the number of calories he will burn in workouts on each day of the first week of the quick start, total them, and divide the sum by seven to get his average daily calorie burn. Note that the calculators on this Web site generate more accurate estimates than some others because they allow the user to enter average speeds for runs and bike rides, which affect calorie burning. Here are the numbers for the first week of Sean's quick start:

MONDAY: Rest day.

Zero calories.

TUESDAY: Run 15 minutes easy + 4 x 30 seconds hard up steep hill, jogging back down for recovery, + 15 minutes easy.

Sean's average pace for easy running is 7:40 per mile, or 7.8 mph. His estimated pace for 30-second hard efforts on level terrain is 5:00 per mile, or 12 mph. It so happens that these 30-second hard efforts are uphill, so he will run somewhat slower, but that doesn't matter; because he's working against gravity, his rate of energy expenditure will be the same as if her were running faster on level ground. Finally, Sean estimates that he will recover with about 90 seconds of easy jogging at 9:00 per mile or 6.67 mph after each hill interval. Add all this together and you get a 38-minute run in which the 206-lb. Sean will cover roughly 4.63 miles and, according to the calculator, burn approximately 712 calories.

WEDNESDAY: 20-minute run + 1-circuit strength workout.

At his easy pace of 7:40 per mile, the 206-lb. Sean will burn about 408 calories in the warm-up run. A single-circuit strength workout comprising 10 exercises takes about 20 minutes to complete. He selects "circuit training – general – minimal rest" from the Web site's list of activities, enters his weight and the duration of the workout, and gets an estimate of 248 calories burned. So Sean will burn a total of 656 calories in this day's training.

THURSDAY: Easy 40-minute run + 1 x 10-second hill sprint.

At his easy run pace of 7:40 per mile, Sean will burn 816 calories in the main part of this workout. His sprint pace is roughly 17 mph. He will burn about 6 calories in one 10-second sprint at this speed. So his total energy expenditure for this workout is 822 calories.

FRIDAY: Cycling power intervals.

This workout features 32 minutes of easy riding plus 2 minutes of maximum-intensity riding. Sean estimates he will average the equivalent of 18 mph on an indoor bike for the easy riding and 33 mph for the sprinting. According to the bicycling calculator on racingweight.com, at 206 lbs. he will burn about 648 calories in this workout.

SATURDAY: Same as Wednesday.

656 calories.

SUNDAY: Easy 1-hour run.

At 7:40 per mile, Sean will burn 1,224 calories in this run.

In the first week of his quick start Sean will burn 4,718 calories. That works out to an average of 674 calories per day.

Now it's time to calculate Sean's BMR.

$$66 + (6.23 \times 206) + (12.7 \times 75) - (6.8 \times 38) = 2{,}043.48$$

Rounding this to 2,043 and dividing by 24, we find that Sean's BMR is 85.1 calories per hour. He sleeps roughly 8 hours every night, which makes for a total of approximately 681 calories burned during sleep.

To calculate Sean's BMR throughout the day, we have to take into consideration the fact that he has a nonphysical job and little time outside of training for exercise. When we multiply his hourly BMR (85.1) by 1.15 (refer to the table on p. 66), we get a total of 97.9 calories burned per hour outside of exercise.

To determine the number of hours of nonexercise activity in Sean's day, we must subtract his sleep time and average daily exercise time in the quick start from 24 hours. Including the additional 20 minutes of running Sean will do in the low-volume running plan, he will exercise 35 minutes (or 0.6 hours) per day, on average. And we already established that Sean averages 8 hours of sleep each night. That leaves 15.4 hours in the day. At 97.9 calories per hour, this means that Sean burns roughly 1,508 throughout the day, outside of exercise.

Sean's daily calories add up to a grand total of 2,863 as follows:

Exercise (.6 hours)	674 calories
BMR (8 hours)	681 calories
BMR nonexercise (15.4 hours)	1,508 calories

Subtract the 400-calorie deficit from this and we get a daily energy intake target of 2,463.

Remember that the quick start protein target is 30 percent of total calories. Thirty percent of 2,463 calories is 739 calories. Since there are 4 grams of protein per calorie of protein, Sean will aim to consume 185 grams of protein daily in his quick start.

STEP 5. CREATE MEAL PLANS

Like all of us, Sean has fairly regular eating habits that must serve as the basis of his quick start eating habits. There are two key challenges he will face in modifying his existing habits to meet the standards of the quick start. First, as a sales professional who works in the field, Sean is often on the road—literally—at lunchtime, so he will have to plan ways of finding restaurant offerings that meet his needs. I would suggest he start by choosing a few specific "go-to" items at popular chain restaurants he likes. The second challenge Sean will face is that his wife, Jocelyn, does much of the family's cooking, so he will need to make his quick start needs known to her so she can prepare appropriate dinner menus. That's not a big challenge; it just requires a little communication.

Here is a sample one-day meal plan that hits Sean's calorie and protein targets. It includes a lunch from a popular chain restaurant. It also reflects Sean's need for a morning cup of joe, accommodates his lactose intolerance by including a soy protein shake instead of a whey protein shake, and makes room for the evening glass of beer that Sean (like his brother!) considers no day complete without.

SAMPLE MEAL PLAN FOR SEAN		
DIET	TOTAL CALORIES	PROTEIN CALORIES
Breakfast wrap (1 ½ servings); strawberries; coffee	2,466	820 (33%)
Soy protein shake		
Burrito with chicken, black beans, lettuce, salsa, and guacamole from Chipotle Mexican Grill (no tortilla chips, which Sean would normally eat); water (source: chipotle.com)		
Apple		
Salmon, brown rice, snow peas (1 ½ servings); light beer		

As I stated in Chapter 5, it is not necessary to plan every meal and snack before beginning your quick start. If you are a born planner and you want to list every meal and snack, feel free, but if (like Sean) you're not, don't sweat it. Some amount of planning is necessary, though. I've encouraged Sean to make short lists of staple breakfasts, snacks, and lunches that he can eat routinely and trust to keep him on track toward his calorie and protein targets through the first two-thirds of the day. His dinner menus can then be more varied and spontaneous. I've coached him to always include a lean protein source as a centerpiece and keep the overall quality high, with vegetables and whole grains typically rounding it out. By keeping track of his calorie and protein intake before dinner, Sean can easily reach (and not exceed) his daily calorie and protein quotas with his dinners by looking up their calorie and protein contents and setting the portion sizes accordingly.

STEP 6. TRACK PROGRESS

The rest is execution. Weigh yourself on a scale with body-fat monitoring capability at least once a week. You can track your numbers as often as every day if you so wish, but if you do, bear in mind that daily fluctuations are less meaningful than weekly trends. (It's not uncommon to gain a few ounces or a pound from one day to the next within a week in which one or two pounds are lost.)

Sean's a bit of a numbers geek (he's the kind of guy who checks his stock values daily, sometimes hourly), so I know he'll have no trouble with this piece. I did, however, have to buy him a body-fat scale to use in his quick start. I'm such a good brother!

AFTER THE QUICK START

The best time to complete a quick start is immediately before you begin training for a race or race season. Let's suppose your next big race is an Ironman 70.3 triathlon and you're going to devote 16 weeks to training for it, perhaps competing in one or two shorter triathlons along the way. Your quick start should begin either four to eight weeks before day one of your Ironman 70.3 training plan or 20 to 24 weeks before your Ironman 70.3 event, depending on whether you choose a four-, six-, or eight-week quick start.

The point of transition between your quick start and your next training cycle is a critical juncture, because your nutrition and training habits will change. To make this transition smoothly, you need to make sure those changes don't occur too abruptly. On the training side, you will presumably reduce your strength training, increase your sport-specific endurance training, and replace the key workouts of the quick start (short intervals and prolonged fat-burning workouts) with different key workouts that are appropriate to the base-building period of the race-focused training cycle. Don't make the mistake of suddenly increasing your endurance training. You can avoid this by including a volume of endurance training within your quick start that appropriately anticipates the volume of endurance training you intend to do at the start of the training cycle, and also by planning a training cycle long enough to allow for a gradual ramp-up to your targeted peak training volume.

On the nutrition side, you will need to make two important changes as you transition from the quick start to your training cycle. First, you will cease to maintain a target calorie deficit and resume eating according to your appetite. Second, you will reduce your protein intake and increase your carbohydrate intake. Fear not; returning to eating by feel will not cause you to regain all the fat you lost, if you eat according to the five steps of the Racing Weight system as described in Chapter 2 and in my previous book, *Racing Weight*. After all, you are an endurance athlete. Nor will eating less protein and more carbs undo your progress if you use Table 2.3 on page 24 to keep your carbohydrate intake in line with your needs, as determined by your new body weight and training volume. What these changes *will* do is ensure that your body is well fueled for your training, so that you get the most you possibly can from the training. At the same time, you can make continued progress toward your racing weight, if necessary, even as you prioritize progress toward your race goals.

Always remember that for the endurance athlete losing excess body fat is a means to the end of racing better, not an end in itself. Resist any temptation to stray from the quick start protocol and the Racing Weight system for the sake of losing weight faster—for example, by trying to maintain your quick start calorie deficit through the training cycle. First of all, it probably won't work. Athletes who eat too little while engaging in heavy endurance training usually experience a metabolic slowdown and a decline in workout performance that cause them to lose less weight, not more. And even if it does work, it will hurt rather than help your racing. Most endurance athletes are pretty good at allowing time to earn the rewards they seek, and if you are more than several pounds heavier than your racing weight, you'll need to call on that patience to get where you want to go. This includes my brother, Sean, who dropped 11 pounds in his quick start and is now working on the last six as he trains for his next—and perhaps his best—marathon.

ABOUT THE AUTHOR

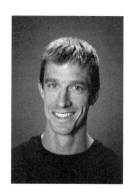 Matt Fitzgerald took up writing when he was 9 years old. He became a runner two years later after running the last mile of the 1983 Boston Marathon with his father (who, of course, ran the whole thing). More than a quarter century later, Matt is still running and writing—mostly about running. He has authored or coauthored more than 20 books, including *RUN: The Mind-Body Method of Running by Feel*, and written for numerous national publications and Web sites, including *Outside* and *Runner's World*. Currently he serves as a senior writer for Competitor Group, whose properties include *Triathlete*, *Inside Triathlon*, and *Competitor* magazines. His special expertise is endurance sports nutrition. He wrote *Racing Weight: How to Get Lean for Peak Performance* and *Performance Nutrition for Runners*, has been a consultant to several sports nutrition companies, and is a certified sports nutritionist. Visit the Racing Weight Web site: www.racingweight.com. Matt lives in San Diego with his wife, Nataki.

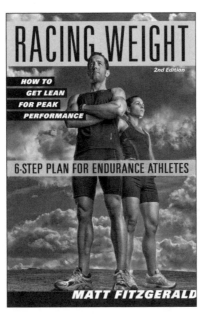
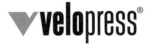